*Ri

Rigged: How Insurance Ruined Health Care

Rigged: How Insurance Ruined Health Care

RIGGED: HOW INSURANCE RUINED HEALTH CARE

By Ralph Weber
With Dave Racer

Alethos Press - St Paul MN
Division of DGRCommunications, Inc.

Rigged: How Insurance Ruined Health Care

ALETHOS PRESS
Div. of DGRCommunications, Inc.
1536 Barclay St, Ste A-1
St Paul MN 55106

Rigged: How Insurance Ruined Health Care
(Previously released as: *MediCrats: Medical Bureaucrats that Rule your Health Care*)

ISBN Print Version
978-0-9849552-4-4
ISBN eBook
978-0-9849552-5-1

Copyright - 2011, 2013, and 2017
      Ralph F. Weber and Dave Racer

All rights reserved. No reproduction in whole or in part in any form is authorized without written permission.

Readers may cite any information with correct attribution.

http://www.medicrats.com
http://www.ralphweber.com
http://www.howinsuranceruinedhealthcare.com
http://www.daveracer.com
http://www.alethospress.com

Third Edition - New Title

Testimonials

"Taking our country back is going to mean getting our arms around our own healthcare. But to do this, people need to understand how the health "insurance" system contributes to destroying health care. In this book, Ralph Weber reveals how "middlemen" rob individuals of their money and threatens their health. Thank you, Ralph Weber, for showing us how we can get better care for far less than the $3.1 trillion we now spend each year."

– Dave Chase
Health Rosetta Institute, CEO and Cofounder

"Ralph Weber's analysis and description of the U.S. health care system is timely. He clearly documents how the third-party payment system not only interferes with the doctor-patient relationship, but also drives up the price of care. The solutions he offers are realistic, and necessary."

–Ming Wang, MD, PhD, CEO, Aier-USA;
Director, Wang Vision 3D Cataract & LASIK Center.

"Read this book and you will understand why ObamaCare has resulted in higher costs and reduced access to health care. More importantly, Ralph Weber shows how the free market and the return of price signals is the only hope we have to return to a rational health care market."

– John Cerasuolo, President
ADS Security, Tennessee

Rigged: How Insurance Ruined Health Care

"Ralph Weber does an excellent job of showing the pending disasters of health care if we continue under the current delivery and finance models. Using simple, real-world examples, he demonstrates the inherent contradictions of recent health care legislation. Fortunately, Mr. Weber offers a way out of the maze with an alternative that refocuses health care on patients, not bureaucrats...harnessing the power of markets to create a patient-centered health care system that cuts through the waste and bureaucracy that dominates health care today."

– Wayne Brough, PhD: Chief Economist and
VP of Research at FreedomWorks

"I consider Ralph my "go to" guy when I have a question. Having his understanding of the issues organized into a printed format is an invaluable resource, especially in this era of health care reform and with the prevalence of misinformation that abounds."

– Lee Kurisko, MD
Practicing physician, Author:
Health Reform: The End of the American Revolution?

"There cannot be a person on this planet that believes in MediBid more than I do! What you created gave me my life back when I had been 'Hung Out to Dry' by my big insurance company and by a big hospital. Before I found MediBid, I had spent more than two years trying to get a total hip replacement and was at a point that I was basically crippled. MediBid allowed me to find one of the TOP surgeons in the country, and the procedure went perfectly as planned."

–Perry Hunt
Huntington Beach, CA.

Rigged: How Insurance Ruined Health Care

"Ralph Weber has found a niche in a health care system gone awry by faulty federal government policy and in so doing, has gained insights and facts, were they better known and understood, would lead to a completely different policy direction from the current trajectory. This is essential reading for anyone who considers himself or herself a health care expert."

– Byron Schlomach, PhD
Director of State Policy - 1889 Institute

"Ralph Weber addresses the most significant flaw in our current healthcare system – insensitivity to healthcare pricing. His analysis is comprehensive. Price insensitivity is directly linked to the third-party payment system foisted on our nation soon after World War II. After all, if it's someone else's money, why should I care what it costs? Ralph's prescriptions for change are exactly what our nation needs. Read this book! Heed its instructions! And join the grassroots movement to alter the healthcare payment model as we know it!"

– Dale Bellis B.A., M.A., D. Min.
Liberty HealthShare℠ Executive Director

"This book is a necessary counterbalance to the disinformation constantly being fed to us by those pushing for government medicine."

– Lee Merritt MD, Orthopaedic Surgeon
Past President of the
Association of American Physicians and Surgeons

Rigged: How Insurance Ruined Health Care

"Doctors are supposed to be diagnosticians. Politicians are misdiagnosticians. But it is Ralph Weber who has provided the unequivocally correct diagnosis for what ails our sick medical care system. Now it is time for us individuals to ignore the politicians and follow Ralph Weber's wise therapeutic suggestions."

– John Hunt, MD
Author of *Assume the Physician*,
Speculator, and *Drug Lord*

"Ralph Weber has been a longtime thought leader on consumer empowerment in health care. He doesn't just think deep thoughts, but has been in the arena putting the ideas into practice. This book will bring you up-to-date with the real world and get you ready for the cutting edge – which has little to do with the latest machinations spilling out of Washington, D.C."

– Greg Scandlen
Healthcare Reform Leader, Author
Myth Busters: Why Health Reform Always Goes Awry

"Ralph Weber is one of the more creative, results-driven consultants with whom I have ever had the pleasure of working. He is able to quickly assess a situation and make recommendations that best fit the client."

– Jacqueline St. Hilaire - D'Alessandro
Past President
Texas Association of Health Underwriters

Rigged: How Insurance Ruined Health Care

This book is dedicated to our families.

Rigged: How Insurance Ruined Health Care

Rigged: How Insurance Ruined Health Care

TABLE OF CONTENTS

TESTIMONIALS	v
DEDICATION	ix
FOREWORD	xiii
Lee Kurisko, MD	
PREFACE	xv
John Goodman, PhD	
MEDICRAT DEFINED	1
SHORT, BUT NECESSARY INTRODUCTION	3
CHAPTER 1	5
Regulating Your Health	
CHAPTER 2	19
Unions, Price-Fixing and the AMA	
Milt Friedman Was Right	
CHAPTER 3	35
With Health Care, Politics Reigns	
CHAPTER 4	51
Moaning and Muttering from	
Health Care Addictions	
CHAPTER 5	73
Defeating Competition	
CHAPTER 6	91
Chargemaster Charade	

Rigged: How Insurance Ruined Health Care

CHAPTER 7 ---------------------------------- 103

    How PPOs Prevent Transparency and Increase Your Cost

CHAPTER 8 ---------------------------------- 121

    Financing Health Care

CHAPTER 9 ---------------------------------- 133

    Health Insurance as Insurance

CHAPTER 10 --------------------------------- 149

    How "Insurance" Ruined Health Care

CHAPTER 11 --------------------------------- 167

    Reference-Based Payment

CHAPTER 12 --------------------------------- 181

    Health Cost Sharing Options

ABOUT RALPH WEBER -------------------------- 189

ABOUT DAVE RACER --------------------------- 191

ORDERING BOOKS ----------------------------- 193

Rigged: How Insurance Ruined Health Care

FOREWORD
By Lee Kurisko, MD

When Ralph informed me that he was going to write a book on health care policy, I could not have been more pleased. Ralph is a treasure trove of knowledge on this subject. Although I have published a book on health care reform myself,[1] I consider Ralph my "go to" guy when I have a question. Having his understanding of the issues organized into a printed format is an invaluable resource, especially in this era of health care reform and with the prevalence of misinformation that abounds.

Ralph and I are both Canadians living in the United States because of the deficiencies of health care in our homeland. He left because of difficulties accessing the quality care that he needed for himself and his family. As a physician, I left because I could not deliver the standard of care that I thought was appropriate due to the constraints imposed by Canada's government-controlled health care system. We did not know each other in Canada.

Through the wonders of the internet, a mutual interest in the failings of health care in both Canada and the U.S. and more than a touch of serendipity, we met while living in the United States. Though we lived in different states, we had innumerable phone and email conversations about health care. We both share the fundamental belief that the problems that we have seen both in Canada (relatively high cost, poor access and poor quality) and in the United States (very high cost and an unaffordable expansion of public programs) can both be traced to the excessive involvement of government in the delivery and financing of health care. Such an idea is not immediately obvious but will become eminently clear in this book.

---

[1] Kurisko, L., MD. *Health Reform: The End of the American Revolution?* Alethos Press, St. Paul, MN. 2009

Rigged: How Insurance Ruined Health Care

Reforming health requires action. Ralph, being a man of action, established "MediBid.com: The Marketplace for Medicine." MediBid.com is an internet-based interactive web portal for buying and selling medical goods and services. MediBid.com cuts directly to the chase of what health care needs and is a powerful platform whereby a free market for health care services can flourish without the intrusion of third-party MediCrats. The prices that health care consumers have obtained with this portal have been very reasonable; a far cry from the massively inflated prices that are so common from facilities functioning exclusively in the government-created third-party payment system.

The United States has painfully discovered it cannot afford the tens of thousands of pages of bureaucratic legalese and regulation that sprang out of the Affordable Care Act of 2010. Once again, and most likely for years to come, we will contend with continuous new reforms. This book reveals how this continuing onslaught of legislation confers neither affordability nor protection upon anyone, except the MediCrats.

All sides of the political spectrum passionately believe that access to high quality health care is of paramount importance. The difference of opinion lies in how that is to be achieved. The knee jerk response of many (myself included until a decade ago) is to believe that the problems we see in health care are best solved with more government involvement. The argument that Ralph makes is the counterintuitive assertion that less government is the answer. In fact, he also shows how health "insurance," supposedly designed to alleviate cost and increase access, is doing just the opposite. This may not seem immediately obvious but will be by the time you complete reading this invaluable contribution to the health care debate.

Lee Kurisko MD FRCPC, is the Chief Medical Officer – www.mediBid.com, a board certified radiologist and Board Member – Consulting Radiologists Ltd.

PREFACE
By John Goodman, PhD

For the last 100 years, government intervention in the health care has resulted in the complete suppression of normal market forces. As a result, almost no one in the medical marketplace ever sees a real price for anything. Employees never see a real health insurance premium. Patients never see a real price for office visits and procedures. Doctors never receive a real price. They receive money based on reimbursement formulas instead.

As a result of the lack of accurate price signals, almost everyone in health care faces perverse incentives. When they act on those incentives, they do things that make costs higher, quality lower, and access to care more difficult than what otherwise would have been. Because patients pay only a fraction of the cost of their care, their incentive is to overconsume. Because doctors see employers and insurance companies as their clients, their incentives are to maximize against reimbursement formulas rather than provide their patients with low-cost, high-quality care. In the absence of prices that clear markets, we rely on rationing by waiting and other non-price barriers to care – obstacles that especially impede access to care for the lowest-income patients.

The health reform act that many called ObamaCare made all these problems worse. Costs are higher; quality may be slipping; and access to care is becoming more difficult because of this Rube Goldberg piece of legislation.

Fortunately, Ralph Weber's book arrives just in the nick of time – at the very moment that health reform is rolling through Congress and state legislatures. After summarizing the history of government interventions in medical care programs, including like Medicare and Medicaid, he shows how each of these well-intentioned efforts actually made things worse. He then makes the case for a free market for health care. He details the problems with recent and current reforms and predicts an upward spiral of prices along with reduced access and a lower quality of care. He observes that modern health insurance is not real insurance. Instead, it's a prepayment for the conception of health care.

Ralph coined the term "MediCrat" to describe the people in power that get to decide how your health care is delivered and paid for: the AMA, unions, Congress, insurance companies, the Centers for Medicare and Medicaid Services. He is blunt about the impact of MediCrats who arbitrarily set reimbursement rates: where no one knows the real cost of care. The market can't efficiently allocate resources if the prices it reacts to are artificial and inevitably wrong.

It is tempting to see this situation as futile, but free markets and entrepreneurship are hard to permanently suppress. Ralph is the architect of a new service, called MediBid.com, that connects patients and providers. Patients who need surgery can log in and, for a nominal fee, receive bids from several different surgeons. The patient then makes a decision based on the hospital's reputation, quality, and price. Ralph's goal is to free doctors to compete on price and to create domestic medical tourism. This will drive down costs for patients and improve the quality of care as well.

I'm grateful for this incisive book, and I'm glad to see Ralph's market-based solution to so many of our current problems.

John C. Goodman is President of the Goodman Institute for Public Policy Research, a Senior Fellow at the Independent Institute, and author of several widely acclaimed, independent books, including *A Better Choice: Healthcare Solutions for America*, and the award-winning, *Priceless: Curing the Healthcare Crisis*. *The Wall Street Journal* and the *National Journal*, among other media, have called him the "Father of Health Savings Accounts."

Explanation of Timeliness

Health care and insurance systems are always in transition. The same is true of laws and regulations related to health care. As we write this book, it is current, but we recognize that many details and facts will have changed after publication.

The 2010 legislation passed by Congress is commonly referred to as the Patient Protection and Affordable Care Act of 2010 (PPACA). The PPACA represents both bills passed by Congress in March 2010. Together, they are referred to as the Affordable Care Act of 2010 (ACA). We use the term ACA in this book.

Once the Republicans took control of Congress and the Presidency following the 2016 elections, lawmakers promised extensive health care reform. We have had a peek at what to expect, but this new round of reforms will not be complete at the time we write this book. We have, however, had the advantage of reviewing a great deal of what the GOP is and will be proposing. Because of this, we are convinced that despite their best efforts, health insurance is still ruining health care.

Rigged: How Insurance Ruined Health Care

They called the Affordable Care Act "Health Care Reform" but knew it meant trying to fix health "insurance" and move regulatory control to Washington, D.C. We have since watched the ACA self-destruct.

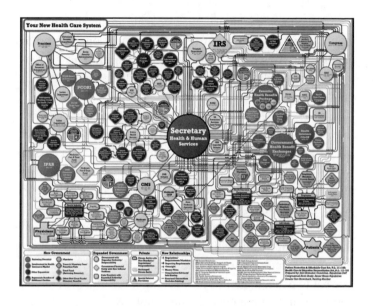

Health care finance is a complex economic system, made more complex by the ACA.

MediCrat:

MediCrat: noun. Medical Ruler

    A health care bean counter working for a government or regulatory agency, a large health plan/insurance company, or medical provider whose primary task is to control the health of a nation's residents and the payment systems allowed to cover health services. The MediCrat approves or disapproves procedures and prices of medical care and sets rules determining utilization of the same.

    Medi is short for medical; *crat* comes from the Latin root word *cratia* – to rule, and the Greek word *kratos* – strength.

    A MediCrat is a person usually with an accounting or cost containment background, appointed by a government official, a third party payer of medical care, or a medical provider who is tasked with reducing the use and price of medical procedures, durable medical products, or prescription medicines.

    MediCratic: adjective. A system in which a single or team of MediCrats dictate procedures and policies applied to the provision or payment of health care services, products, and medicines.

    MediCrats are the inevitable and expensive by-product of a health delivery system in which insurance is expected to pay for all or most of medical and mental health care. MediCrats are "rent seekers," whose expense is underwritten by money spent for insurance paid by others who have little or no control over costs charged by medical professionals.

Rigged: How Insurance Ruined Health Care

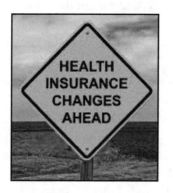

Short, but Necessary Introduction

Health care and insurance systems are always in transition. The same is true of laws and regulations related to health care. As we write this book, it is current, but we recognize that many details and facts will have changed after publication.

The 2010 legislation passed by Congress is commonly referred to as the Patient Protection and Affordable Care Act of 2010 (PPACA). The PPACA represents both bills passed by Congress in March 2010. Together, they are referred to as the Affordable Care Act of 2010 (ACA). We use the term ACA in this book.

Once the Republicans took control of Congress and the Presidency following the 2016 elections, lawmakers promised extensive health care reform. We have had a peek at what to expect, but this new round of reforms will not be complete at the time we write this book. We have, however, had the advantage of reviewing a great deal of what the GOP is and will be proposing. Because of this, we are convinced that despite their best efforts, health insurance is still ruining health care.

Rigged: How Insurance Ruined Health Care

CHAPTER 1

REGULATING YOUR HEALTH

The most powerful form of control a government can have over an individual is to regulate his or her health. This is precisely why the government, powerful medical unions, health insurance companies, and the massive health care provider organizations and Pharma have been battling for a piece of the health care pie for so many decades. For the government to control its people, its goal is to establish a MediCratic system where medical rulers have authority to decide when, where, and how health care will be delivered.

Until Congress passed Medicare and Medicaid in 1965, the United States had refused to sponsor federal government-run and government-paid health care. However, by creating these two national government health care programs, whether it meant to or not, Congress began taking the lead on how Americans received their health care. Congress created the MediCrat. Medicare especially, has come to dictate to a large extent, 1) how individuals of all ages receive health care, 2) the types of care they can access, and 3) the price they pay for it.

Congress extended MediCrat control over health care from just public programs to private health care when it passed the HMO Act in 1973. Since then, every year Congress has increased MediCratic control over both public and private health care. By 2015, the system that Congress established had pushed health care spending to $3.1 trillion. Yet, the irony is that Congress fretted about nearly 46 million "uninsured" people to such an extent that it felt Washington, D.C. knew best how to overhaul health care for everyone.

From having very little to do with health care in the early 1960s, today, Congress essentially sets national health care priorities and determines its regulations. Because of its political meddling, finally, in 2010 Congress took a giant step toward controlling all of U.S. health care. On March 23, and March 30, 2010, Congress passed the two new laws we now know as the Affordable Care Act of 2010 (ACA). Since then, we have seen how the ACA has caused massive spikes in the cost of health insurance and reduced an individual's choices of physicians and medical facilities – with one exception.

> Nearly 16.7 million additional individuals were enrolled in Medicaid and CHIP in February 2017 as compared to the period prior to the start of the first Marketplace open enrollment period (July - Sept. 2013).[1]

We have seen that the ACA asserts MediCratic power to regulate individual lives and the affairs of all the professionals and businesses that serve individual medical needs. America's founding fathers would roll in their graves if they knew this had happened. Some people, however, claim the founders had passed a similar law.

---

[1] Staff, Center for Drug Evaluation. "February 2017 Medicaid and CHIP Enrollment Data Highlights. Medicaid.som, (February 2017)." https://www.medicaid.gov/medicaid/program-information/medicaid-and-chip-enrollment-data/report-highlights/index.html

Did Congress Set the ACA Precedent in 1798?

On July 16, 1798, Congress passed the "Act for the relief of sick and disabled seamen."[2] The new law required ship owners to pay 20 cents per month per employed seaman to the U.S. Secretary of the Treasury. The act required the President to use the funds, as needed, "…to pay to hospitals or other proper institutions now established in the several ports of the United States…"[2] Is this the same thing the ACA did when it mandated that every United States' resident must buy health insurance? Does it speak at all to a precedent whereby Congress can assert control over individual health care? No.

It helps to understand why Congress passed the law. Seafaring carried huge physical risks, and without American ships carrying goods back and forth across the ocean, U.S. foreign trade could not have existed. Everyone in the United States was engaged in building their new country; agriculture took precedence over much of all domestic commerce. Yet, to prosper, the new nation had to engage in robust trade with foreign nations. This required ships and able men to operate them.

The "seaman law' recognized the fact that seamen played a pivotal role in the success of foreign trade. The Constitution had given Congress the right to regulate trade with foreign nations. Everyday citizens to ship owners and the merchants they served recognized the value of and relied on trade. Trade created much-needed wealth for the shipowners, merchants, and for the new nation. The trade in question related to the 1798 Act, however, dealt with foreign nations, and did not apply to trade between individuals or businesses within the colonies. Nothing in the law mandated

---

[2] Chapter 94: An Act for Relief of Sick and Disabled Seamen. U.S. Congress. July 16, 1798. Signed by President John Adams.

that anyone, other than ship owners and seamen, do anything or own insurance.

The Fifth Congress, by passing the 1798 Act, required the seaman to pay part of their earnings into a pool of money in advance of an illness or injury. Unlike the ACA, the 1798 law never levied a general tax on Americans, nor did it require that non-seamen also must own insurance. In fact, the 20 cents did not buy health insurance: The funds simply sat in the U.S. Treasury until the President paid the bills of one of the seamen who had paid into the account. It worked like a self-funded workers' compensation pool for a tiny sliver of America's working people.

FACT: The 1798 Act was not health insurance, and Congress never tried to apply it to anyone but seamen involved in foreign trade. No case for health care reform today can be built on it. Having been given the authority to regulate foreign trade, it protected the men who enabled the means to that trade.

Meanwhile, Across the World

Unlike the United States government, some foreign nations began building national, government-run financing systems to pay medical bills of their citizens. Germany's employer-based, universal health insurance system began in 1883. Japan launched its national system in 1928. The United Kingdom followed in 1948. "Medicare in Canada is a government-funded universal health insurance program established by legislation passed in 1957, 1966 and 1984."[3] But in the United States, at least until Congress passed

---

[3] *Making Medicare. The History of Health Care in Canada*, 1914-2007. Retrieved on July 7, 2011. http://www.civilization.ca/cmc/exhibitions/hist/medicare/medic01e.shtml

Medicare and Medicaid, the government had not taken any such action.

In the U.S., insurance companies initially avoided writing medical insurance. In 1919, a trade magazine, *The Insurance Monitor*, wrote:

> ...the opportunities for fraud [in health insurance] upset all statistical calculations.... Health and sickness are vague terms open to endless construction. Death is clearly defined, but to say what shall constitute such loss of health as will justify insurance compensation is no easy task.[4]

It is amazing to see that 90 years ago, private companies that were asked to risk their own money, knew that the argument about "what shall constitute loss of health" could not be answered easily. Today, the same argument rages, but government put itself in the place of providing answers, and the answers are driven by politics, not financial markets.

"In the first quarter of the twentieth century, then, health insurance was little used and, for that matter, remained little needed."[5] Less than 300 hospitals existed across the nation. Doctors rarely had skills that exceeded those of "Barber Surgeons." A U.S. "health care system" as we think of it today, did not exist.

Birth of the Blues

In 1929, businessman "Justin Ford Kimball...offered a way for 1,300 school teachers in Dallas to finance 21 days

---

[4] Random History. "In Sickness and in Health: the History of Health Insurance." Retrieved on June 17, 2011. http://www.randomhistory.com/2009/03/31_health-insurance.html.

[5] Blue Beginnings. BlueCross BlueShield Association. Retrieved on June 29, 2011. http://www.bcbs.com/about/history/blue-beginnings.html.

of hospital care by making small monthly payments to the Baylor University Hospital."[6] This led to creation of Blue Cross, a way to raise money from individuals to prepay hospital care. Still, it would not be proper to call this hospital insurance in the sense we think of it today. It did, however, find a way to pay hospitals for the increasing number of patients for which they provided care.

Meanwhile, the federal government started providing grants to various communities and charitable groups to build and expand hospitals (today there are more than 5,000). More hospitals meant more health care was being provided.

President Franklin Roosevelt promoted universal health care during his first term, but failed to convince Congress. However, he did get Congress to pass the Social Security Act in 1936. "Physicians were concerned that the contemporary social security legislation would lead to compulsory health insurance that would be heavily regulated and devastate patient choice and their relationship with physicians."[7]

Eventually, the American Hospital Association urged its physician and surgeon members to form their own prepaid plans, which came together under the name of Blue Shield in 1939. These new Blue Shield plans would help physicians and surgeons be surer of receiving payment for hospital-based and major medical services. Other physician services, like routine office calls or physicals, were still paid in cash (or perhaps, with a dozen eggs or a side of beef).

In the early days, what we now call "health insurance" was called accident and sickness insurance, since those were the expenses it was meant to cover. In other words, hospitals created Blue Cross to ensure they could get paid for services

---

[6] See Note 4.
[7] See Note 4.

provided, and physicians and surgeons created Blue Shield so they could be paid for services they performed.

During World War II, Congress imposed a wage freeze on employers. As a result, employers began offering health insurance as an employment benefit, in lieu of higher wages. Thus, by imposing its will on private employers, Congress upset the common employment incentives provided by salaries, wages, working conditions, and industry. Employers adapted, and used health insurance as the incentive when trying to hire and retain good employees. Congress went along with it, because it still understood that in the United States, businesses placed a high value on productive labor. President Calvin Coolidge had said, "After all, the chief business of the American people is business. They are profoundly concerned with producing, buying, selling, investing and prospering in the world."

The long term effects of employer-provided health insurance are still felt today, but not because of how it started. Over time, employer-provided health insurance has grown into a cornucopia of tax-favored benefits including, after 1973, comprehensive medical insurance that pays for routine care. Thus, a simple $1.40 a month group health insurance premium in 1965[8] has grown to $536 a month, or more, in 2016 (for single coverage).

Congress meddled again

In 1954, Congress continued to manipulate the ownership of health insurance when it changed the IRS code to allow employers to receive a tax deduction for the health insurance benefits paid to employees. This meant that neither the employer nor the employee paid income or social secu-

---

[8] Johnson, H. (2007). Harlan Johnson Insurance Agency. Receipts on file. Pequot Lakes, MN.

Why health care inflation outpaces cost of living

In 1954, when Congress decided to allow employers to deduct health insurance as an expense, it changed how people purchased health care. Employers soon realized they could provide a great benefit for employees and save money at the same time – save money for both parties. It works like this:

An employer decides to spend $1,000 on a health insurance plan instead of paying the employee $1,000. Both parties save money.

The law allows the employer to deduct 100 percent of the $1,000 from company income – the employer pays no income or payroll taxes on the $1,000. The $1,000 costs the employer $1,000.

The employee pays no income or Social Security tax on the $1,000. After 1965, the employee also paid no Medicare tax on the $1,000. The $1,000 buys $1,000 in benefits.

If a modern-day employer pays the employee $1,000 in salary instead of providing a health benefit, it might cost the employer as much as $1,250 (payroll taxes, workers compensation, unemployment insurance, and other payroll-related cost). It is true the employee will receive $1,000 more compensation, but the employee will pay Social Security, Medicare, and income tax on it. Depending on the employee's income tax bracket, the $1,000 in compensation might result in as little as $600 in the employee's pocket.

Since an individual policy is not tax deductible for an employee, if an employer desires to provide one it might cost the employer as much as $2,000 before tax. This would leave the employee with $1,000 in take home pay with which to pur-

> chase a policy, compared to $1,000 for a $1,000 employer funded policy.
>
> After the 1954 tax code change, employers shifted annual increases in compensation away from salary, and toward tax effective benefits. Health plans became richer and richer, while pay increases became smaller. This increase in health care spending caused health insurance companies to develop more costly plans, which in turn drove up healthcare utilization and healthcare inflation, while moderate pay increases kept general inflation lower.

rity taxes on the cost of medical or hospital insurance. This new tax law made it more attractive for employers to shift money away from pay raises and toward more health insurance benefits and this triggered an unending increase in inflationary health spending. The insurance of that day, however, remained mostly limited to paying hospital-related and major medical costs. No one owned "insurance" to pay for routine care.

In a Supreme Court case, decades before the ACA passed, the Court ruled that health insurance did not qualify as an object of Commerce. In Paul v. Virginia, the Court ruled "…that insurance contracts 'are not articles of commerce in any proper meaning of the word' as they are not objects 'of trade and barter,' nor are they 'commodities to be shipped or forwarded from one State to another, and then put up for sale' ")."[9]

Then Congress tried an end run around the Supreme Court by once again, attempting to regulate insurance. In 1944, the Court, in United States v. South-Eastern Underwriters, did a pivot, and gave the federal Congress the authority to regulate insurance under the Commerce Clause.

---

[9] Racer, D. (2011) "A Condensed Version of Judge Roger Vinson's Ruling Overturning the Affordable Care Act of 2010." DGRCommunications, St Paul, MN. May 2011. P. 3. http://www.freemarkethealth care.com

Like today after the passage of the ACA, the states protested, and as a result, Congress passed the McCarran-Ferguson Act in 1945. This left the regulation of medical and hospital insurance in the hands of state regulators. State regulation of medical and hospital insurance, eventually called health insurance, did not change until Congress gave the Federal Secretary of Health and Human Services overarching control over it when it passed the ACA in 2010. In 2017, Congress intends to offer states the opportunity to apply for waivers that would reduce some federal control over state regulation.

Finally, Congress encouraged a new medical entitlement mentality when it passed the HMO Act of 1973, thus giving preference to HMOs over traditional private health insurance plans. By the mid-1970s, the march toward government-controlled, MediCrat-managed health care entitlements had begun to flourish, and eventually, grew into the Affordable Care Act of 2010, which is neither affordable nor could it provide care in the years to come. Hence, even more federal attempts to reform health care continue to be debated.

We can conclude a great deal from this brief history:

- First, pooling money to pay for unforeseen medical and hospitals bills started out as a rational idea promoted by physicians, surgeons, and hospitals to make sure they received payment for their services.

- Second, Congress passed laws hoping to enhance the continued productivity of employees – providing a tax break to employers that provided coverage to their employees.

- Third, when Congress passed Medicare and Medicaid, it put the government in direct competition with Blue Cross, Blue Shield, and the scores of other companies that paid medical and hospital claims. Once Congress passed Medicare and Medicaid, people with private insurance started demanding the same "benefits" being paid for with their tax dollars in those programs. Congress obliged with its 1973 HMO Act.

- Since the time that Congress overstepped its constitutional authority in the 1940s, and ever since, the role of politics in the provision and payment of the cost of health care has grown to the place where it is today – run by an army of MediCrats: Politics drives health care.

From no insurance in 1919, we moved to voluntary private coverage. Employers used health insurance to protect their employees' health; this was a logical means of protecting their investment in people. At the same time, Congress, however, with its wage restrictions and tax law changes had interfered with the free market for labor. Today, Congress has involved itself with every minute detail of our health care and insurance systems.

Until 1965, we did it without the politicians

By the late 1950s, hospitals stood in communities across the country, from large cities to rural towns and counties. Poor people received much of their care from facilities provided by local communities, churches, temples and other religious institutions. Every community seemed to have a St. Andrews, St. Johns, Catholic or Jewish Hospital. Counties also provided hospitals and clinics to serve the needs of poor people. As the number of hospitals grew, so did the number of health insurance policies, which incentivized increased usage of medical services to "fill the beds" of these expensive new facilities.

Physicians billed patients directly and collected from them, and expected as many as 20 percent of their patients to trade in something other than cash – or perhaps receive free care. Prior to 1966, society expected people to provide for themselves, and even with health care, they did it. This is the attitude that had prevailed from America's beginning.

U.S. health care evolved rapidly during the 20th century. It could not have done so unless Americans believed in the value of individual work and earning one's own way. For a limited time, that was not true of our first settlers, when some people felt that they had special privileges that isolated them from work.

Most of the first colonists died within three years of landing at Jamestown, Virginia in 1607. The problems presented by the disease-riddled place where they chose to settle would have been tough enough, but their lives were made even more miserable by several stubborn aristocrats. Those aristocrats thought that others should do the work, and that they were entitled to position and leisure at the expense of the lower class. While the farmers, craftsmen, and artisans went to work, the aristocrats sat back, expecting others to provide their needs. Everyone suffered.

After the "starving winter" of 1609, of the 500 settlers who had come to the place [Jamestown], only 60 still survived. The fact that the aristocrats had refused to work had placed an added burden on everyone and their arrogance contributed to this needless death.

Captain John Smith's edict, "He that will not work shall not eat," became the byword of those 60 survivors. The hundreds of thousands of colonists who followed later put into practice this same idea...[10]

Today, more than 125 million of men and women still get up every day, go to work at full-time jobs, and earn their keep. Unfortunately, millions of other Americans think that they are entitled to receive health care at other people's expense. This new entitlement mentality grew out of the actions of Congress since 1965. This attitude led us to the Affordable Care Act, a government plan that attempted to provide taxpayer subsidized health care for as many as 68 percent of our population. Ironically, we have seen much of the same MediCratic arrogance in Washington, D.C. during the passage of the ACA as we saw exhibited by the aristocrats in Jamestown. Once again, as in that day, this arrogance will cost many lives as the rationing begins, and wastes trillions of dollars before that. It is as though the aristocrats of the 17th century passed their values to the MediCrats of the 21st century.

Americans have come to see that the ACA threatens America's future as much as did the lazy inaction of those early Jamestown aristocrats. Once again, Americans demand that Congress pass reforms, still relying on the misconception that what they are buying is health "insurance." Ironically, this never could have happened without the complicity of the "union" to which most physicians belonged so many years earlier.

---

[10] Racer, D.; Dattilo, G. (2006) *Your Health Matters: What you need to know about U.S. health care.* Alethos Press LLC. St Paul MN. P 10-11.

Rigged: How Insurance Ruined Health Care

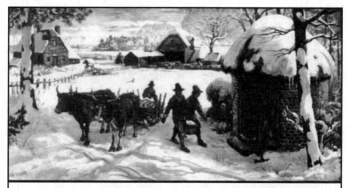

Within five years of settling in Jamestown, more than 500 people had died. In many cases, death could have been avoided if everyone had adopted the edict, "He that will not work shall not eat." Society benefits most when its members take responsibility for themselves.

Chapter 2

Unions, Price Fixing, and the AMA: Milton Friedman was right

Milton Friedman, the esteemed economist, describes the American Medical Association (AMA) in his classic book, *Capitalism and Freedom*. Friedman labels the AMA as the "strongest trade union in the United States." Then he proceeds to document how the AMA vigorously restricts competition. The AMA, Friedman says, uses its Council on Medical Education and Hospitals to control the supply of Medical Care. The Council uses its power to restrict the number of medical schools and approves how many applicants those schools may accept. In this way, the AMA limits the supply of physicians. This sounds much like how OPEC's Oil Cartel quadrupled the price of oil when it withheld output during the 1970s.

Because the AMA directly affects the reimbursement rates physicians receive for medical care, in essence, the AMA is directly negotiating physician wages. This is the customary process controlled by a trade union. And like unions, it guarantees that low quality doctors will be paid the same rates as the best.

Across the country, school districts face the daunting task of managing budgets which are subject to union contracts. Union negotiators have built expensive and generous benefit systems for teachers, but perhaps more important are the rules related to salaries and teacher tenure. Because of these union contracts, it is more difficult for most school districts to terminate the employment of lower quality teachers, and they are faced with paying all teachers the same salaries, not based on quality but on longevity or educational achievement.

Although physicians do not specifically belong to unions, their incomes are subject to a similar kind of regulation as are teachers' salaries. For physicians, the regulations come from MediCrats at the Centers for Medicare and Medicaid Services (CMS) and the American Medical Association (AMA).

CMS is a federal agency funded by tax dollars with broad duties that are felt across the health care system. Of all its duties, perhaps the one felt the most, is CMS' setting of the Medicare reimbursement rate paid to physicians, hospitals, and other medical providers. CMS uses at least 13 different reimbursement systems to determine what and how it will pay.

Medicare employs a complex coding system to reimburse physicians, hospitals, and other medical providers. For medical and surgical procedures, CMS uses Current Procedural Terminology (CPT) codes. "The ranges of CPT codes goes from 00100 through 99499 and include approximately thousands of CPT codes. There are in some cases, some two digit modifiers that may be appended when it is appropriate."[1] By adding two digits, the number of potential codes increases dramatically. The AMA produces and manages the CPT codes, in 2011, according to their website, earning

---

[1] Cagle, C. (2009). *ICD-9 Codes and CPT Codes*. Associated Content from Yahoo! http://www.associatedcontent.com/article/1538545/icd9_codes_and_cpt_codes.html?cat=5. Retrieved on June 29, 2011

nearly $78 million a year in royalties for their use. In this, AMA is acting like the unions in that the CPT codes result in price-fixing of reimbursements for all physicians and hospitals who accept Medicare – and private insurance.

Private insurance companies use the Medicare reimbursements from CPT codes as the foundation upon which they set their own reimbursement rates. Health insurance companies negotiate reimbursement rates for medical services as a percentage they are willing to pay above the Medicare rate. In this manner, AMA and CMS have colluded to control the price of health care for private and public programs.

Yet, as a way to spend our hard-earned tax dollars, CPT code rates function like a pre-negotiated fee schedule from a union. A physician in practice for 30 years with a medical degree from Harvard gets reimbursed the same as the physician just hired by the same clinic. Physicians consistently report that Medicare and Medicaid reimbursements at best only meet the raw cost of providing services – usually even less.

To earn enough money off this CMS/AMA regulated system, clinics must reduce quality, and one of the most common methods is limiting physician time with patients – to five minutes or less per office call. The clinic can provide more patient time, but to afford it, must use a Physician Assistant (PA) or a Nurse Practitioner (NP) to provide the medical care that should require the physician's attention. The clinic can allot more time with a PA or NP than with the physicians, as they cost the clinic less. The more codes that can be entered into the bill and the more bills that can be sent, the more revenue the clinic can generate, but at less cost per transaction. In some ways, older, more experienced physicians cost the clinic more since they spend more time with the patient, whereas young new doctors spend less time, and order more tests, making them more "profitable."

(We do not write these facts to condemn the physicians or the clinics – or the PAs or NPs. Medical clinics and hospitals are not immune to the realities of time and the cost of staying in business. The clinics and hospitals must adapt or go out of business. If any service provider is paid $10 for a service which costs $15 to provide, he or she must make a choice between reducing quality, or adding billable options to the service.)

The CMS/AMA's price-fixing scheme is a fundamental problem in our health care payment system. It serves to distort the prices an individual should actually pay to receive care. The CPT coded pricing scheme, as it too often grossly underpays actual physician cost, forces them to inflate their billing price to the private insurance companies. The insurance companies, in turn, "discount" the billed prices (we discuss this insidious system elsewhere) and pay only a portion of them. Ironically, the individuals that pay the most for health care under this system are the people without health insurance who must pay cash for services, except those using MediBid. The current CMS/AMA price-fixing scheme creates cost-shifting from the public to private individuals, leaving perceived prices high.

The AMA strongly endorses the use of health insurance, of course, since it is the principle method by which their members are paid (that, and government health plans). It's why physicians and surgeons urged the creation of Blue Shield and Blue Cross – so they could be paid in cash, rather than trading for eggs or a side of beef.

The AMA also strongly endorsed the provisions in the Affordable Care Act of 2010 that forced every American to enroll in a health plan, whether with private health insurance or on a taxpayer-funded plan. During its June 2011 national conference of delegates, the AMA reiterated its support for the ObamaCare individual mandate. The issue of the constitutionality of the individual mandate was settled by a Supreme Court decision in 2012. The Supreme Court said the ACA mandate is constitutional, labeling the mandate a tax. Congress it ruled, has the right to tax.

When the AMA endorsed the individual mandate, it is akin to unions using the power of government to require "prevailing wage" laws that force government units to pay top dollar for construction contracts. Every payer must play in the same employment pool, under the same rules, with little ability to negotiate.

The Affordable Care Act also required the formation of Accountable Care Organizations (ACOs). These act like Health Maintenance Organizations (HMOs) on steroids. HMOs are notorious for their perverse incentives to physicians that less care is good because it saves money. Congress believes it will be easier to control cost by herding physicians, surgeons, and other medical providers into ACOs – large organizations – and then use the leverage of these ACOs to deliver services more efficiently. Local physicians and surgeons fear they will be unable to work unless they sign up under an ACO. This is similar to another union tactic. Unions hate "right to work" laws that force their members to compete with non-union employees for jobs and contracts. ACOs, like unions, do not want to have to compete with hundreds of small competitors.

The AMA, like unions, prefers government enforcement of "membership" through its 2011 endorsement of the individual mandate, price fixing by its CPT codes, its cozy relationship with CMS, and by organizing physicians into ACOs. Does it, however, benefit the health care consumer?

In 2017, as Congress considered "repeal and replace" of the Affordable Care Act, the AMA stubbornly insisted that the new Health Care Reform Act would leave more individuals uninsured.

By 2026, it was estimated that 52 million Americans would have lacked health insurance, 24 million more than under current law. On March 22, 2017, the AMA wrote to House Speaker Paul Ryan and Democratic Leader Nancy Pelosi to inform the Congress that the AMA was unable to support "legislation that would leave health insurance coverage further out of reach for millions of Americans."[2]

The AMA Trustee Board quotes from the highly creative estimates of the Congressional Budget Office to justify their fear. The AMA clearly suffers from the "Stakeholder Syndrome"[3] in which their "seat at the table" and need to remain in control of their mission clouds their thinking about new health care legislation that could benefit everyone – that could, in fact, stop a stampede to government-run, single payer health care.

Here is an example of how the AMA/CPT code system has hurt consumers – this example is common to medical providers across the United States. In Minnesota, the Medicare reimbursement set by the CMS/AMA price-fixing scheme sets the reimbursement rate at $542 for an MRI. The Medicaid price for the same MRI is $367 ($175 less for the same service). The insurance company for a person with a health plan would reimburse the clinic at about $695. Yet, if an individual called and asked for the cash price the clerk would quote them about $1,250, or might discount it 25 percent to $935. So for this one service, we see a price swing

---

[2] Harris, Patrice, MD. (2017) *Report of the Board of Trustees – 6-A-17*. The American Medical Association. Washington, D.C. https://www.ama-assn.org/sites/default/files/media-browser/public/hod/a17-bot06_0.pdf P 2.

[3] Beecher, L.; Racer, D. (2017) *Passion for Patients*. Alethos Press, St. Paul, MN.

of as much as $883 – from $367 to $1,250. The MRI clinic might lose money providing services to Medicare and Medicaid patients, and then attempts to make it up by charging more to people with insurance or who pay cash.

Total knee joint replacement reimbursed by Medicare using CPT codes is about one-fifth of the national average billed price. The same type of result is seen looking across the broad spectrum of CPT-based reimbursements. One would think that since the effects of the CPT codes are so pervasive, they would be open to public inspection. To make CPT codes appear to be transparent, the AMA has published a catalog linked to its website, but, "The AMA reserves the right to limit your access to the File and may limit the number of searches and/or the number of CPT codes per search."[4] The AMA has made its CPT coding system opaque, and not transparent, by severely restricting public access to them. This also allows the AMA to charge tens of millions of dollars for the use of the CPT code look-up service.

CMS also allows some access to CPT codes on its massive website, but its complexity is enough to make a mature, experienced researcher weep. Certainly, the CMS/AMA partnership has made this scheme so complex as to render it useless to a health care consumer – perhaps it is on purpose.

Price-fixing is an artificial way to set the cost of health services. As it pays Medicare providers too little, it forces the price higher for individuals who receive health care from non-government sources. As a result, the clinics, hospitals, physicians, surgeons, pharmacists, medical device suppliers and the entire army of service providers must inflate their bills for private-pay patients. Is there a way to resolve this problem?

If the U.S. health care system could operate in an open, competitive free market with price competition and

---

[4] https://catalog.ama-assn.org/Catalog/cpt/cpt_search.jsp

transparency, it is likely we would see prices drop to meet actual cost with an appropriate margin for profit to the medical provider. In a free market environment, a good, experienced physician would be able to charge more for his or her time than what would be charged by a rookie doctor, and quite a bit more than a PA. More importantly, in a free market system, the patient could choose whether to see the MD or the PA.

In a free market, instead of the AMA/union-like market of today, perhaps the MD and PA would design systems to work together to maximize health care quality at an acceptable price. If health care operated more like other professions, the consumer would expect to pay more for a specialist than a generalist: you expect to pay a CPA more to do your taxes than a book keeper. Small businesses often employ bookkeepers for routine work, but see the CPA for more complex tasks and tax work. If accounting operated like health care, you might never see the CPA, and be forced to rely on a bookkeeper to offer critical financial advice.

When the CMS, working with the AMA, imposes price restrictions on them, physicians and hospitals are left without recourse but to serve Medicare patients at a loss and in return, soak the private pay patients. Since the Medicare contract is voluntarily entered into by the physician – he or she is not forced to sign up with Medicare – maybe that is the real fair market price and they are overcharging the rest of their patients. The fair market price of any product or service is the most the payer is willing to spend for it and the least the provider is willing to accept as payment. If physicians are willing to accept Medicare reimbursements as acceptable payment, maybe that is the price they should ask of everyone else. (One other choice exists for now: physicians can refuse to provide care to Medicare and Medicaid patients, and indeed, this is a growing trend. Once it becomes overwhelmingly serious, look for Congress to mandate that every licensed physician must accept government-covered patients.)

The sorry thing is that taxpayer and private insurance policy holders finance this inefficient pricing system. Medicare's costs are paid through a payroll tax. Medicaid's costs are paid through general taxes. Private insurance is paid by individuals or their employers (and if by employers, health insurance costs are passed along in the price of goods and services). Because the self-insured population is often billed at "jacked up prices," it often makes medical care less affordable for them. If they fail to pay their medical bills, the providers report the losses at the full price, making their loss seem greater than it might really be.

Another group of individuals are self-insured by choice. These might be wealthy people, or others that do not believe in insurance, but can pay their own way if needed. Some communities still band together to pay for the medical cost of their members. Some religious groups have faith-based exemptions under the ACA, since they share medical costs – we devote a chapter to these health care cost sharing organizations in this book. All of these, however, end up paying an inflated price for health care in traditional hospitals and clinics. No one escapes paying the inflated price of health care services (unless they have access to market-based tools or the ability to hire private physicians on their own).

The CMS/AMA price-fixing scheme inflates the price of health care. One might think that it keeps prices lower for Medicare recipients, but that fact cannot be determined. Why? The entire health care system must comply with the complex rules imposed by MediCrats that result from the government reimbursement system. There is no way to determine the efficiencies a private market could create while operating under these government rules. There are some hints, however, and these options need to be explored. The fact that procedure costs for Medicare recipients are often lower than costs usually results in one of several outcomes:

1. Medicare recipients have a difficult time finding a doctor to work for "less than cost."
2. Medicare recipients may receive lower quality care, seeing a Physician Assistant instead of an MD.
3. Medicare recipients receive extra services which may not be needed in order that the doctor's office may receive enough to cover costs.

Many physicians today are turning to cash-only medical practices or to concierge medicine. By so doing, physicians who refuse to sign up with Medicare or refuse private insurance payments find they have greatly reduced their overhead expense. They can practice without a large, expensive support staff and less costly compliance advisors – the MediCrats' power over them is diminished. Their attention is spent on patients, instead of trying to comprehend and administer a complex administrative office.

Cash-only physicians must price their services so that patients understand their bills – and can afford to pay them. Imagine the value patients could enjoy if they received all their health care in a system where market forces – the interaction between patients and their physicians or hospitals – determined the price, not the CMS/AMA MediCrats. Imagine if medical bills were easy to understand!

When Congress passed the Affordable Care Act, what we now refer to as ObamaCare, in 2010 they told us the idea was to repair the elements that drove health care prices higher. Instead, ObamaCare reinforced and exacerbated the status quo; actually, it made it worse. By relying on the police power of the federal government, increasing MediCratic power to enforce a whole new regime of top down management, ObamaCare moved 180 degrees away from consumerism. Instead of putting patients and doctors in charge of treatment decisions and able to directly negotiate prices, ObamaCare gave that responsibility to MediCrats and 15 unelected members of the Independent Payment Advisory Board (IPAB), and scores of new and costly federal agencies. The third party payer system has been continuously manipulated by Congress from its beginning. Forcing more people into MediCratically-approved health plans while decreasing deductibles will only drive costs up further.

ObamaCare's IPAB was designed to serve the same role as the union bosses at the National Education Association, or the international union bosses at the Service Employees International Union. The IPAB "bosses" would have determined which medical and surgical procedures should be covered, and directly or indirectly, the price of medical care. The IPAB MediCrats would set the "work rules" for medical practice through implementation of so-called "practice guidelines" or "evidence-based medicine." No one questions that doctors need guidelines – it's why they go to medical school and why they keep reading and learning. When those guidelines, however, come from a powerful, unelected political entity – the IPAB – they serve more as edicts: edicts that resemble union work rules.

ObamaCare attempted to solve the wrong problem by funding third-party paid health care for tens of millions more Americans. It did this at the expense of fixing a more important problem: the high and increasing price of medical and hospital care. Fixing the cost of insurance without allowing markets to function, however, is futile.

> **FORMULA: THE COST OF HEALTH INSURANCE**
>
> ASSET PURCHASED
> x UTILIZATION
> + OVERHEAD
> + TAXES
> + PROFIT
> COST OF INSURANCE

At the end of the day, no matter how you slice it, the cost of insurance or any kind of financing scheme is based on the underlying cost of the purchased asset or service, times utilization, plus the overhead costs, and profit.

ObamaCare tried to attack the cost issue by declaring it would pay less to physicians and hospitals. Congress, however, did not actually let this happen: Each time the reduction in Medicare reimbursements came up, Congress canceled the cuts (here again, the AMA "union" steps in to apply political pressure). Without the cuts, however, Medicare and ObamaCare could not survive – they will bankrupt the system.

Congress has made another attempt to control physician income through the 2015 Medicare Access and CHIP Reauthorization Act – MACRA. While MACRA repealed the previous fee-setting program, its new formulation relies on an incentive payment system determined by federal MediCrats. Time will tell if physicians do better under MACRA, but for certain, MACRA ignores and disrupts price and demand economic signals.

With ObamaCare, Congress passed laws intending to reduce the Medicare reimbursement schedule (and every other payer schedule which is based on it) by 41 percent over the next decade. The Congressional Budget Office, in predicting the cost of ObamaCare, based its spending projections on the assumption that these cuts would occur. ObamaCare attempted to add coverage for millions more people who were "uninsured," reduce deductibles, and decrease the cost all at the same time without gutting those reimbursement rates – this is not possible. Perhaps Congress should have asked a better question: How will senior citizens be able to find competent, compassionate medical care if doctors' reimbursements are cut by 41 percent at the time that the MediCrats force increased administrative compliance costs on medical providers?

ObamaCare also relied on dictating the terms of the "Medical Loss Ratio (MLR)." The MLR is arrived at by dividing health insurance premium into two parts: one part pays medical claims and the other part pays all the other cost associated with insurance (customer service, marketing, management, claims handling, plus taxes and so forth). Congress arbitrarily declared that under the ACA, insurance companies must pay 80 percent of each premium dollar for claims, and no more than 20 percent for everything else – on individual and small group health insurance plans. (For large group plans, Congress said 85 percent had to go toward claims, with 15 percent for everything else.)

Congress meant to cut the cost of health insurance using the MLR, but the ACA did nothing to change incentives to hold down total health care spending. Spending is directly related to how often a person uses a service – utilization. If the cost of an office visit is $1, utilization wouldn't much matter. At $100, however, utilization does matter. So before we talk about all the other factors Congress tried to use to hold down spending, we need to tackle 1) the cost of the underlying service or asset – the medical care; 2) the utilization incentives, such as low deductibles or the disconnect from the price: these are what really drives health care spending.

If the average health plan premium is $500 per month, then the MLR allows 20 percent ($100) for overhead. If an insurance company takes steps to reduce premium by increasing co-pays and deductibles, by cutting mandates, and by reducing reimbursement rates, and the premium fell to $250, it would only leave them with $50 for overhead. This, of course, makes no sense. The overhead costs do not go down – they either remain constant or increase. Actually, the MLR provides an incentive for insurance companies to increase premiums, thereby also increasing their 20 percent overhead share.

If the insurance company charges all people $10,000 a year in premium, at the end of the year, it must have spent at least $8,000 on medical care for the entire group. Otherwise, it must return money to everyone. If your group chooses to become healthier, or ignores going to the doctor for routine health care, the insurance company will pay out less in claims, and must return more money. It will also have less left over for overhead when it is forced to adjust its insurance premium rates. Compare this to life insurance where the insurance company hopes you live a long life, and meanwhile, invests your premium dollars for decades: this is where they earn their money. This keeps premiums affordable for life insurance companies. For health plans, however, the insurance company needs you to consume services so it can collect increasingly more in premium – if it does not, their 20 percent overhead share will fall.

If you pay $1,000 a month for health insurance, you think you should use it to get value from your expenditure. If you do not file a claim, or use medical care, you feel you were robbed.

Rigged: How Insurance Ruined Health Care

If you buy auto insurance, however, you don't rush home and figure out how to spend it – and the cost is probably more like $1,000 a year. When you purchase homeowners' insurance, you hope you will never have to use it. With health insurance, however, you almost feel obligated to use it. Why? Not necessarily because you need medical care, but because the insurance system incentivizes you go to doctors, especially with the new MLR as described above. Think about it. Would health insurance cost rise or drop if people only went to doctors for illness? Some health plans, however, have someone call you to beg you to use the coverage. The health insurance company MediCrats call this preventive care, and lobby Congress and federal MediCrats to cover dozens of procedures. Then insurance reimburses 100 percent of the cost, but not without raising your premiums to pay for it.

Remember that the hospital association created Blue Cross and then expanded the number of hospitals, so if we don't "use" our health plans, how will they pay for all of these facilities?

ObamaCare ran 180 degrees away from market-based health insurance incentives. ObamaCare attempted to resolve the pricing problem by severely limiting the private practices of physicians and surgeons, and imposing rules on hospitals and other medical providers.

The AMA, with its coding system and its partnership with CMS, is a key enforcer of this union mentality. The AMA's paid membership is likely less than 15 percent of practicing MDs – the figure is obscure, but a huge number of practicing physicians avoid active membership. "Very soon, the membership of the AMA will be below 10 percent of practicing physicians," said Jane Orient, MD, Executive Director of the Association of American Physicians and Surgeons. Yet through the CPT coding system, the AMA controls nearly all physicians in the same manner as unions with less than 11 percent of employees as members still manage to maintain a stranglehold on the private economy.

To resolve the health care pricing problems, Americans need market reforms where individuals hold bargaining power rather than the AMA, insurance companies or government. We must break the AMA/CMS stronghold on the status quo. We need to reduce and, as much as possible, eliminate the power of the federal government and its CMS MediCrats.

A free market in health care can break the stranglehold of the AMA and CMS MediCrats. As you continue reading you will find how this can be accomplished.

CHAPTER 3

WITH HEALTH CARE, POLITICS REIGNS

We showed you in Chapter 1 how health care became so political at the national level, but we did not mention state-level politics. Long before Congress passed the ACA in 2010, politicians across the country were making decisions about local health care and insurance. Remember, in 1945 Congress passed the McCarran-Ferguson Act to make sure that states remained in control of private health insurance. When we say states have control, however, we recognize that control is exerted by the political processes.

The political process in each state works its will on members of state legislatures (called assemblies in some states). State Representatives and Senators who like holding office listen to the constituents that are most likely to help them win elections. Legislators rely on lobbyists for information, strategy, ideas, money, and votes.

Politics is a contact sport played by people with strong opinions and beliefs. They fall, broadly, into two camps. Conservatives tend to support laws that reduce the power and reach of government. Liberals tend to support laws that increase the power and reach of government. Conservatives tend to believe that individuals know how to manage their own money: By this, the entire economy will grow and everyone will benefit. Liberals, on the other hand, tend to believe that government can manage money better than individuals: Good government, a liberal believes, means taxing and spending more so that everyone will "benefit."

In her classic book, *Atlas Shrugged*, Ayn Rand labels big government believers as "looters" and the people that live off government programs as "moochers." Rand, along with most conservatives, believed that private ownership of money that is invested by individuals brings the greatest benefit to society. On the other hand, looters and moochers steal away the productive capacity of individuals. In the liberal world, everyone loses, except the bureaucrats who run government programs.

Conservative legislators tend to rely on marketplace mechanisms to control health care and insurance cost, and try to hold down taxes that go to pay for health care. Liberals tend to use government as a tool to provide and pay for health care, even as it increases taxes to pay for these expanded services.

Legislators seldom create something new. Instead, they pick up where the previous legislators left off – playing the hand they were dealt. When legislatures met in 1946, after Congress had passed the McCarran-Ferguson Act, they wrote new laws about regulating health insurance. In some states, conservative legislators wrote only a few laws that were general in nature; in others, there were many specific laws that were broad in their applications. After that, each year, new legislators picked up the previous version of the law and built on it – seldom does a legislature dismantle a law, although it may modify it toward more liberal or conservative principles.

Once Congress restored states' power to regulate health insurance (McCarran-Ferguson), instead of asking, "Do we want our state to regulate health insurance?" legislators asked, "How do we want to regulate health insurance."

Once states started, they tended to increase insurance regulation, not decrease it.

With health care, lawmakers have always have had a hard time taking away a benefit or program or plan once the legislature has added it to the law. Instead, legislators tend to expand benefits, programs, and plans, to reach more voters – people.

James Payne, PhD, wrote in his book *The Culture of Spending: Why Congress Lives Beyond Our Means*, that for every 144 individuals that testify to Congress, only one asks that a program be discontinued, or funding cut back. The others come with their hands out, asking for increased budgets and program expansions. Until the Tea Party revolts during the 2010 election, Congress (and most state legislators) seldom heard the message to cut or eliminate programs.

During the time of the slow, normal process of growing laws beyond their original intent, President Lyndon Johnson unleashed the Great Society in 1965. Johnson declared war on poverty and as a result, created dependency on government which we now call the entitlement mentality. In its 2014 report on the Fiftieth Anniversary of the War on Poverty, the Heritage Foundation stated:

> Since that time, U.S. taxpayers have spent over $22 trillion on anti-poverty programs (in constant 2012 dollars). Adjusted for inflation, this spending (which does not include Social Security or Medicare) is three times the cost of all military wars in U.S. history since the American Revolution.[1]

Millions of Americans now vote for politicians based on the monetary and program benefits they will receive or

---

[1] Sheffield, Rachel, and Rector. "The War on Poverty After 50 Years." The Heritage Foundation. Accessed May 12, 2017. /poverty-and-inequality/report/the-war-poverty-after-50-years.

lose, rather than what strengthens the country or state. Nowhere is this more evident than with health care.

To be reelected, expand, expand

There is an old saying that people get the kind of government they deserve. A corollary is that politics is run by those that show up. If the voters, activists, and lobbyists that show up are constantly begging lawmakers for an increasing number of benefits, then we end up with a health care system in which everyone feels entitled to everything they want at someone else's expense. The dirty secret, known by every socialist and capitalist politician, is that conservative citizens on the whole want nothing to do with politics – they must work for a living. Liberal citizens, on the other hand, know that without politics, they will lose control – and their jobs.

When it comes to health insurance, "more" is translated into dozens of mandates on health plans. For instance, the battle is raging across the country over mandating coverage for the treatment of autism. "Twenty years ago, autism affected somewhere around 1 in 2,000 children. Today, it affects 1 in 110 children…autism prevalence has increased dramatically over the past 20 years…an estimated 600%."[2] No one knows why this has happened.

When parents of autistic children come together, hire a lobbyist, and begin demanding that legislators require (mandate) that state insurance companies add autism coverage, it is hard to resist. Public relations, telephone campaigns, post cards, letters, and a flood of emails assault lawmakers. The personal stories pull at their heartstrings and make the evening news. Some witnesses accuse legislators

---

[2] Halladay, A.; Rosanoff, M. (2011). *Evaluating Change in Autism Prevalence: Change We Can Believe In?* Autism Speaks Official Blog. Retrieved on July 9, 2011. http://blog.autismspeaks.org/2011/02/03/s-evaluating-change/. Feb. 3, 2011.

of heinous indifference. The primary concern for the lawmaker, of course, is whether voting for or against this mandate will result in reelection or expulsion.

(Political pressure on lawmakers by potential voters is one of the greatest positive features of our republican form of government. Elected officials are supposed to respond to voter pressure, and in its purest form, it works for the betterment of everyone. The cards, however, are stacked against those who believe in limited government for the simple reason that they tend to be busy taking care of their families, not lobbying at state capitals for more benefits.)

Each new mandate on insurance increases the cost of monthly premiums, and monthly premiums are how we finance health care. The more mandates, the greater the cost of coverage. There is a secondary effect that is more serious: Each time a mandate is added, the use of medical care increases. Why? Someone else is paying for the care, not the individuals who have the medical condition. Parents of autistic children, who might find less costly ways to help their children, will spend tens of thousands of dollars if their health plan covers treatments – with someone else's money. That is human nature: and politicians know it. That it is why by 2017, 47 states now mandate some level of coverage for autism.

Average 43 per state

The total number of mandates for all 50 states equals 2,156 – an average of 43 (all references to the number of mandates are drawn from the CAHI report cited below).[3] Idaho has the least: 13. Rhode Island has the most: 69. Each mandate adds cost to insurance premiums. The more man-

---

[3] Bunce, C.; Wieske, J. (2011). *Health Insurance mandates in the States 2010.* Council for Affordable Health Insurance. Washington, D.C.

dates, the more expensive insurance will be, all other things being equal.

How did Rhode Island get to 69 mandates and Minnesota to 64, when Idaho would settle for 13, and Alabama, for 19? Rhode Island and Minnesota are "progressive" states. This means that over the years, each legislature has added more entitlements, instead of reducing or even maintaining the number of entitlements.

Idaho is a very conservative state, as is Alabama. Their former legislatures never added in dozens of mandates, so each new legislature starts with a lower number. Idaho voters are not at the capital demanding more mandates, and apparently, there is no money to organize activist groups and hire lobbyists to pressure lawmakers to add more mandates.

You would expect that if you could buy the same insurance policy in Idaho as you could buy in Rhode Island, just based on mandates, the Idaho policy would cost far less. However, it is more complicated than that.

Ten states mandate coverage for wigs (hair prosthesis). Lawmakers required this because they were sympathetic to cancer patients. Chemotherapy often results in hair loss; mandating insurance payment for wigs for people who lose their hair during cancer drug treatment makes sense to lawmakers in those 10 states. It might add 10 cents to the monthly premium. Any attempt to eliminate the insurance mandate for wigs, however, is met with an emotional backlash by oncologists, cancer patients, and wig makers. Would you want to be the legislator that tells a bald, cancer-laden patient he or she should pay for their wig out of pocket, instead of by insurance?

Wigs are cheap compared to drug abuse treatment, and 34 states mandate coverage for the treatment of drug abuse, which can cost tens of thousands of dollars. So, it is not just the number of mandates, but the potential cost of each that is worrisome.

Connecticut has 59 mandates, while New York State has 52. Connecticut mandates coverage for wigs, but New York does not. Both states also mandate the extremely expense procedure called in vitro fertilization; helping barren women become pregnant. They, however, have different requirements in their mandates and this is another reason health insurance costs more in New York State than in Connecticut.

Teresa Pica-LeRuo, 42, of Connecticut, wanted to have a baby but is unable to conceive naturally. She went to an infertility clinic for help, but, "Pica-LeRuo and her husband said they can't afford in vitro fertilization on their own..."[4]

As a result of the requests of infertile women (and most likely, fertility doctors), Connecticut joined the 14 other states that mandate health insurance policies to offer infertility treatments as a covered benefit. "The legislation...requires most individual and group insurers to cover a lifetime maximum cost of two in vitro fertilization cycles, three intrauterine insemination cycles, and four ovulation induction treatments per patient."[5]

The benefit could cost insurers tens of thousands of dollars per conceived child: "...one round of *in vitro* fertilization typically costs $12,000, and couples often have to try multiple times to become pregnant."[6]

The new Connecticut law at that time, however, denied the infertility treatment benefit to women older

---

[4] Haigh, S. (2005) "Conn. Enacts Law on Infertility Treatment." Associated Press writer, Hartford Courant, September 26 2005.
[5] Ibid.
[6] Ibid.

than 40, like Pica-LeRuo. "Though she wants Connecticut lawmakers to remove the age limit, she is considering changing jobs and moving to New York to get coverage."[7]

If Pica-LeRuo does move, New York residents will bear a financial burden of $12,000 or more to help her become pregnant – and more to cover her pre-natal, delivery and post-natal expenses. New Yorkers, especially those who have never filed a claim, will wonder why their insurance premiums are more expensive than in Connecticut, unaware that it is because the costs of Pica-LeRuo's in vitro treatments and other health expenses must be covered. Pica-LeRuo's medical costs are paid out of that same pool of insurance money.

The question you might be asking is why does health insurance cover in vitro fertilization in any state? The short answer is politics. In New York, the fertility doctors and their patients were able to convince legislators to mandate in vitro fertilization. Fertility doctors believed that forcing insurance companies to cover fertility treatments would give them more patients to serve. The doctors have so far convinced 15 states to go along with this scheme. They have been unable, however, to convince politicians in 35 other states – at least, not yet.

What does this mean for you? Obviously, if you never want to have in vitro fertilization, you would not want to buy insurance in New York State. Idaho would be a better choice, if you could. There are, however, other considerations.

Some other ways politics drives up (or restrains) mandates

All across America a political battle rages about whether men should be allowed to marry men, and women

[7] Ibid.

allowed to marry women. For dozens of years, gay and lesbian activists have been pressing for states to recognize same sex marriage. Then, in 2015, the U.S. Supreme Court, in Obergefell v. Hodges, ruled that states could not prohibit same sex marriages.

Prior to the Supreme Court decision, however, gay and lesbian activists had convinced 18 state legislatures to mandate insurance coverage for "Domestic Partner Civil Unions." In other words, people that opposed same-sex marriage in Colorado were required to pay more for health insurance than their neighbors in Montana who also may have opposed same-sex marriage. At the time, Minnesota, a progressive state, did not mandate coverage for gay couples, but Iowa did. This created the peculiar situation in which neighbors, living within eyesight of each other across state borders, would have different health insurance premium cost – based on the success or lack thereof of folks to convince lawmakers to sanction gay marriage.

Mandatory coverage for same sex couples, then, depended on a political process. The political process is generally won by whichever faction can better rally their troops, raise the money, and bring fear to incumbent lawmakers. This process is clearly not driven by economic market forces, but by sociological preferences turned into political action.

Laws for those who abuse themselves

Alcoholism and drug abuse are a terrible scourge on addicted individuals and costly both in terms of poor health and related medical cost. Society, too, pays for the sometimes tragic results of individuals driving under the influence of alcohol or addictive drugs – and even of prescription medicine. There are, of course, plenty other ways individuals practice behaviors that predictively result in increased medical expenses.

What is a politician to do about obesity? If people eat too much, eat foods that make them obese, and exercise too little, what can Senator Skinny do about it? Sen. Skinny knows that more than half the cost of health care is lifestyle related, and a good portion is because of obesity. Unfortunately, 35 percent – or more – of Sen. Skinny's voters are obese.

Sen. Skinny's solution is to force insurance companies to treat everyone the same for insurance purposes. Instead of relying on individual characteristics (what the insurance industry calls underwriting) Sen. Skinny wants to rely only on age, and even then, Skinny doesn't want 60-year olds (who vote) to pay too much. Sen. Skinny likes the idea of "community rating" and writes a law requiring all insurance companies to use it to determine their monthly premiums. Here is how it works:

Suzy Oversize is 45, and weighs 230 pounds. According to the government, Suzy should weigh 125. Suzy has many health problems that could be alleviated if she lost weight and exercised, but her 5'4" frame prefers resting a lot. Suzy should be paying $800 a month for health insurance, but she chooses not to buy insurance.

Sarah Slight is 62, and weighs 120 pounds, the same as the day she graduated from high school. Other than having children, Sarah has never been sick or hospitalized. Sarah should be paying $200 a month, if insurance was measured only on health history, but pays $400, because of her age.

Samantha Young is 25, and weighs 135. She's relatively healthy, although she has a couple of margaritas every day. She's suffered from a mild form of asthma most of her life. Other than that, she's had very few medical issues. Samantha pays $100 a month for health insurance.

Rigged: How Insurance Ruined Health Care

Sen. Skinny decides to split the difference between Samantha, Suzy and Sarah – using community rating. He convinces his political friends to average out the cost of individual insurance premiums based on their age, not their health status. When Sen. Skinny got his bill passed, and then signed by the governor, Samantha's insurance increased to $175, Suzy's fell to $375, and Sarah's shot up to $525. Suzy is happy.

In some states, politicians fell in love with community rating so that Samantha, Suzy, and Sarah, all pay $435 a month, and Samantha drops coverage. Politicians, however, called Samantha a freeloader, and passed a law mandating that she must buy health insurance – Samantha moved to Idaho.

ObamaCare, and its successors, mandated the use of community rating. The ACA, in fact, limited insurance companies from charging more than three times the premium to older individuals compared to the youngest adults – a 3 to 1 ratio. The only exception was an upward adjustment for tobacco users. Hence, fewer young people purchased the new coverage because its cost had gone up too much. Older individuals, however, may have originally received a premium cost reduction. As a result of community rating, combined with other ACA mandates, the cost of individual health insurance sky-rocketed. New efforts to reform community rating simple spread out the ratio to 5 to 1.

Imagine if auto insurance was sold using community rating. Dan Drunker, who has had three DUI convictions and five serious auto accidents, would pay the same insurance premiums as Sam Sober. Sam has never had an accident, while Dan has had many. Do you believe they should pay the same auto insurance premiums? Thankfully, politicians have not given into such foolishness about auto insurance –

at least, not yet. Yet, this is the same thinking as goes into health insurance community rating.

Remarkably, states use tobacco taxes to pay the cost of many medical programs, including health insurance for children – CHIP. Since the early 1960s, cigarette manufacturers had to place warnings on their packages. Perhaps the modern-day adaptation of this idea is to require tobacco companies to place this label on each pack: "Light one up for the kids." Seriously, fewer people are smoking, and the taxes states rely on are less than they hoped.

The ACA

The Affordable Care Act of 2010 created insurance mandates: It called them essential benefits. The law mandated the following insurance coverage:

1. Ambulatory patient services.
2. Emergency services.
3. Hospitalization.
4. Maternity and newborn care.
5. Mental health and substance use disorder services, including behavioral health treatment.
6. Prescription drugs.
7. Rehabilitative and habilitative services and devices.
8. Laboratory services.
9. Preventive and wellness services and chronic disease management.
10. Pediatric services, including oral and vision care.[8]

---

[8] Section 1302. The Affordable Care Act of 2010.

Rigged: How Insurance Ruined Health Care

No one knew how many mandated benefits would result from these so-called essential benefits. For instance, ambulatory patient services covers most clinical care. Does it mean that everything done in a doctor's clinic will be covered? We could never afford everything.

Imagine if the government MediCrats required us all to own "Food Insurance." If government bureaucrats decided on the essential benefits of Food Insurance, would they mandate chuck steak, filet mignon, or chateaubriand? It probably would depend on the power of the chateaubriand lobby.

If we are to remain a free people, we must be ever vigilant as our elected officials add benefits to win votes.

The ACA gave the federal Secretary of Health and Human Services power to decide the rules about each of these benefits. The rules are managed by MediCrats and subject to ongoing politics for decades to come. Remember, the MediCrats have their own union to protect their programs.

The ACA offered an example of how politics affects the mandates. The ACA required that all preventive care services be paid by insurance at 100 percent of the contracted price. How the Secretary defines the word "preventive" is the key. Congress worried about this, and so specified that the decision had to be made by the United States Preventive Services Task Force (USPSTF). The USPSTF is a longstanding government bureaucracy. It has created various definitions of preventive care, and put them into tables. The ACA said that preventive care, to be paid at 100 percent of price, is any service on list A or B, as recommended by the USPSTF – but it makes one major exception.

> (5) for the purposes of this Act, and for the purposes of any other provision of law, the current recommendations of the United States Preventive Service Task Force regarding breast cancer screening, mammogra-

phy, and prevention shall be considered the most current other than *those issued in or around November 2009*. [Emphasis added][9]

This astonishing paragraph in the new law showed clearly how politics drives health care decisions, not science. The reason for this exception was simple: when the USPSTF issued its report on annual mammograms, the political outrage was heard everywhere. The USPSTF had found that annual mammograms could actually threaten the health of many women, and recommended against annual mammograms. The media exploded with the story that women would be denied mammogram coverage. Within days the politicians began to hear from thousands of angry women, they added language to the ACA so despite the science, women could get their mammograms. This is normal behavior for a politician, but it should not be for a scientist and those whom determine what will or will not be paid by mandatory health insurance.

What will be the next expensive breakthrough

Unless continuous government intervention kills investors' interest in new medical technology, we know that new breakthroughs are just around the corner. Will these new devices, treatments, and procedures be subjected to scientific review, or MediCratic politics? Since 1965, the answer is quite clear: Politics drives medical care.

Many medical device inventors give up when Medicare refuses to cover their device, no matter how much good it would bring, or that might reduce health care spending. The Medicare MediCrats decide, not the marketplace. If the marketplace decided, then the best products at the most reasonable price would be available to the public. MediCrats

---

[9] Section 2713(a). The Affordable Care Act of 2010.

make their decisions based on what the politicians have decided, not the marketplace. Therefore, they inhibit the marketplace from sorting out the good from the bad, the effective from the ineffective, the expensive from the affordable.

We are not opposed to insurance. We are, however, strongly opposed to politics trumping good health care decisions. Health insurance companies have tremendous clout both in Washington, DC and state capitals. The health insurance companies and an army of third party payers, tend to get what they want out of politicians, although it may appear to be otherwise.

The ACA relied upon an individual mandate that required everyone to be covered by private health insurance or a government health plan. To make it work, politicians decided to tax broadly and use tax money to subsidize insurance premiums for as many as 62 percent of the population. This would never have happened except for the complicity of major health insurance companies.

Health Insurance companies understand that the more people who have insurance policies, the more cash insurance companies will be able to invest. They have a vested interest in everyone being forced to own health insurance, but very little interest in holding down health care spending. In fact, just the opposite is true. The more people spend on health care, the more health insurance companies can collect in premium. As explained earlier, the Medical Loss Ratio (MLR) provides insurance companies with an incentive to increase premiums, and increased premiums result from increased health care spending. Without the collusion of health insurance companies and the politicians they seem to own – and with support from the American Medical Association – the ACA would never have passed, at least with an individual mandate to buy insurance. Only voters and health care purchasers can change this.

Rigged: How Insurance Ruined Health Care

Before we can remove the powerful influence of politics from medical care, we have to remove the politicians that favor it. Unfortunately, that task is made far more difficult because we have become used to the entitlement mentality. As Pogo said, "We have met the enemy and he is us."[10]

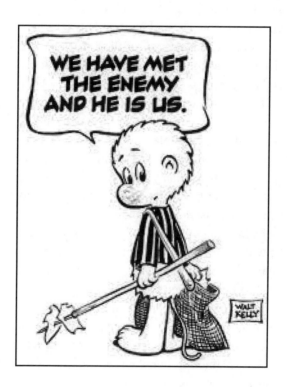

---

[10] Kelly, Walt. *Going Pogo.* 1970 and 1971

Chapter 4

Moaning and Muttering from Health Care Addictions

If you hang around physicians very long you are sure to hear them complain about their reimbursements. Whether it's Medicare, Medicaid, or insurance companies doing the reimbursing, to physicians the third-party payers are at fault.

In contrast, when you take your car to a mechanic, you never hear a complaint about "reimbursements." Why?

The auto mechanic will give you a good faith estimate of the charges to repair your car before the work begins. The estimate is quite specific, and it reflects the mechanic's hourly charge. You can decide whether to go ahead with the repair and pay the mechanic's rate, try to do it yourself, or drive a mechanically impaired car. You never hear the mechanic say, "My hourly rate is too low, I don't get paid enough."

If your auto repairs are covered by insurance or a maintenance contract, it is not unusual for the insurance company to require three written estimates in advance. This is one way the auto insurance companies make the mechanics compete for your business. They realize that competition reduces costs. In essence, MediBid.com reduces cost like this, from competition created by requesting more than one bid for a medical service.

More importantly, the auto mechanic will never fix your car and send the bill to someone else (unless, of course, it is an auto body shop where repairs are covered by insurance). If you agree to have the work done, you will pay for it. In other words, the mechanic does not get reimbursed – he gets paid when the work is done.

Physicians, hospitals, and other medical professionals perform services for you, but are paid by others called "third-party payers" (unless you are either uninsured or have a high deductible health insurance policy). When these "others" pay the medical provider, it is often weeks or even months after the service has been provided before the payment is received. This is why it's called a "reimbursement" – reimbursing the medical provider for services performed long before the patient sees the price.

Often, when the third-party payer finally makes the reimbursement, it is made for a lesser service than was provided. This is called "down-coding." The third-party payer disagrees with the code used on the billing and changes it. Or the payment is based on a CPT code which has a lower reimbursement level. For example, the physician may bill based on the code 99214 at a rate of $138, but be paid $33.68 for code 99213. A routine office visit of minimal complexity is a 99213, while a 99214 is an office visit with moderate complexity. Sometimes doctors are reimbursed even lower based on a "silent PPO." This means that the doctor participates with several payers, and sometimes one of those payers will reimburse based on the lower paying reimbursement schedule.

Rigged: How Insurance Ruined Health Care

The reimbursement payment system used today is the result of hospitals creating Blue Cross, and physicians creating Blue Shield. Physicians and hospitals provided services to people who owned insurance, and waited for payment. When health care was simpler and payments much smaller, it probably was a workable system. Health care, however, is no longer simple and is quite expensive.

Following after the creation of Blue Cross and Blue Shield, hundreds of other companies created their own health insurance policies. Once HMOs became popular, individuals expected to see a physician and pay little to nothing for the service out of their own pocket. It also made it possible to have surgery in a hospital, and recover there for several days, and never pay much at all out of one's own pocket for the service.

Medicare and Medicaid nationalized the idea of direct physician reimbursement for medical and surgical services. It put federal and state government MediCrats in charge of the method and amount of payment for medical services. It is true that in most locales, the reimbursement amount for Medicare-paid services is less than private insurance. It is also true, that in most places, Medicaid pays even less than Medicare.

Insurance companies base their reimbursement payments on Medicare's reimbursement levels. If, for example, Medicare reimburses a primary care physician $60 for a simple office visit, it is likely a private insurance company will reimburse at about $84 (although you may have to pay a co-pay). The percentage varies from insurance company to insurance company, and health plan to health plan. In some places, where there is almost no competition between private insurance companies, Medicare might actually reimburse more than the insurance company.

Therefore, the MediCrats that staff government and insurance company bureaucracies are deciding the price of medical services, not the free market. Yet, medical providers have become addicted to this form of payment. Many, if not most, are scared to death of even thinking of "selling" their services directly to patients. Frankly, physicians, surgeons, hospitals, pharmacies, and all the other medical services that care for patients may complain about the MediCrats' control of reimbursements, but most show by their actions that they prefer this system to dealing directly with patients.

Once individuals enroll in Medicare, they visit doctors more frequently. This could be due in part to their age and the infirmities it spawns, or as some doctors insist, the individual is lonely and a trip to the clinic is a social event. It could also be because the Medicare system really gives the motivation to overuse the system. Whatever the reason, it is a boon to the clinic as it is able to bill Medicare for more services. It is a boon to pharmacies, too, as physicians use medicines to "relieve suffering," conveniently paid by Medicare Part D.

Ready-made business model

Jack Jones graduated from business school with an MBA. Jack owed $200,000 in student loans. While still in college, Jack invented a new medical product. He believed it had remarkable financial potential, and would bring much-needed relief from suffering to thousands of individuals.

After he graduated, Jack spent five years raising money to complete and bring his product to market. All during this time, Jack lived in a one room efficiency apartment, drove a beat up old car, and ate oatmeal, bologna sandwiches, and Ramen noodles. Then he received the phone call he desperately awaited, from his attorney.

Rigged: How Insurance Ruined Health Care

Jack's attorney had persuaded the Medicare MediCrats to add his device to the list of approved durable medical devices. After that, it was only a matter of time when private insurance companies approved his device. Soon after, Jack was able to earn a six-figure income. Over time, Jack became a multi-millionaire. He finally paid off his student loans 20 years after graduation. Unfortunately, jealous of his financial success, many in Jack's community disparaged him as a cold, heartless industrialist.

Janet Johnson graduated from medical school, and then finished her internship and a four-year residency in general surgery. Janet owed $200,000 in student loans.

During her residency, she received a monthly stipend equal to the average income in her area. Janet lived in a simple two-bedroom town home she shared with another resident. It was close to the hospital. She enjoyed gourmet meals, and frequented the nice restaurants nearby.

Three months before Janet finished her residency, a major surgical group in a large metropolitan area offered her a $200,000 base income to join their staff. Within five years, Janet was well established in her community.

Janet bought a large home on a lake, with a three-car garage. Everyone who knew her felt she deserved it and held her in high esteem. No one would disagree, especially her patients. Janet paid off her student loans 10 years after finishing her residency.

Both Jack and Janet are smart people and well-educated. Both eventually earned high incomes. Janet, however, never had to struggle putting together a successful business. Unlike Jack, medical doctors walk into an established practice most of the time. Jack had to build from scratch, and follow good business practices, denying himself many comforts, until he finally hit the jackpot. (Most Jacks never hit the jackpot.)

Rigged: How Insurance Ruined Health Care

Janet never ran the risk that Medicare, Medicaid, and private insurance companies would quit reimbursing her for her services – even if she felt they paid too little. Jack always contended with the reality that at any time, the MediCrats could decide that his medical device was no longer needed.

So, Jack kept on designing and building more medical devices to ensure his financial future (and he started the Jones' Medical Foundation to provide his devices to low-income inner city residents).

This story about Jack and Janet demonstrates the reality that physicians, surgeons, and many who practice medical care on a daily basis never have to face the harsh realities of living without a reimbursement system that is pretty much guaranteed money. Janet, quite frankly, would prefer to worry only about her next patient, not about her next paycheck – and that's how most of us would prefer it to be. She, however, often complains about how much she is reimbursed and the MediCratic control under which she must work.

Through a time-tested, sophisticated network of referrals and third-party payers, Janet's surgical practice can count on a regular patient flow. She does not have to fight for market share as Jack does when another manufacturer makes a device like his.

Jack eventually sold his device company to a huge international corporation. He retired at 55 with hundreds of millions of dollars.

Janet's surgical group signed a contract to belong to the Midwest Accountable Care Organization – MACO. This allowed Janet to let go of all administrative functions, keep working, and earn a great income – even though slightly less than previously.

Eventually MACO agreed to be purchased by a Mega Health Insurance Company – MHIC. MHIC had contracts with hospitals, clinics, and pharmacies across the region. As the payer and provider of care, MHIC's MediCrats were able to deal directly with the MediCrats at the federal Department of Health and Human Services, and Medicare.

Meanwhile, Janet kept doing surgery and being paid well – with reimbursements flowing like oil.

With money comes control

Physicians and surgeons have a legitimate beef with the MediCrats that pay them. With money, comes control. The MediCrats want to tell the physicians how to practice, control the tests they can order, and limit the medicines they can prescribe. This is very frustrating for physicians and their patients – and it does not produce the most efficient, quality health care.

Why, then, do physicians continue to practice under MediCratic control? It is as if they suffer from battered spouse syndrome.

The physician knows that for every service he or she performs, the chances of being paid are greater if the patient has health insurance or is covered by a government health plan. This is a very secure way to do business.

Perhaps the physician's need for security outweighs their desire for practice freedom. It is hard to resist the demands made on a physician by a third-party payer MediCrat when that clerk directly affects your paycheck. Dr. Johnson can complain as much as she likes, but the MediCrat will have the final say. If Dr. Johnson doesn't like it, she can always start a cash-only practice.

Had Janet Johnson become a rural family practice physician in a single-doctor clinic, she would have lived with economic insecurity. At the same time, she may have enjoyed the patient–physician relationship far more than working as a surgeon in a large practice. In her single-doctor clinic, Janet may have even more strongly opposed interference by the MediCrats.

Hospitals, likewise, seem to prefer to work with the MediCrats rather than fight them. Hospitals storm state capitals and Congress with ongoing horror stories about what will happen if reimbursements are cut – or not increased again. Yet, hospitals seem unable to find private market solutions making them financially viable without MediCratic reimbursements. This may stem from the days when hospitals invented Blue Cross to get paid. Perhaps the hospitals – and physicians – have never severed the umbilical cord. This might explain why they continue to play the "chargemaster game," and pay lobbyists to win the sympathy of Congress.

Keeping the cash cow happy

At least since 1965, health care and health insurance have become political issues. Nearly everything is decided by state legislators and members of Congress.

To keep the cash cow churning, the medical provider community makes sure to be well-represented in front of politicians. Politicians, for their part, know that to be re-elected means making sure that constituents are happy. This often means, in terms of health care, keeping physicians and hospitals well fed and on a strict diet at the same time. Politicians need people coming to them asking for favors and there is probably no other industry feeding more often at the political buffet line than the health care industry.

The politician knows that he or she can count on the support of those who are dependent on the MediCratical reimbursement system. It seems not to matter which political party is in control, the medical and hospital lobbyists somehow manage to convince lawmakers to keep the money spigot open, at least enough to survive until the next budget period each fiscal year.

Having old friends helps

Pundits and political consultants often state that Medicare and Social Security are the third rails of politics. This means that any member of Congress that attempts to reform these two very expensive programs can count on political attacks from the gray panthers – so candidates try to avoid saying anything that smacks of real reforms. The gray panthers take their lead from the American Association of Retired Persons (AARP).

In 2015, AARP had operating income in excess of $1.54 billion.[1] Of that, $295.2 million came from dues paid by millions of members. Dues, however, play a minor role in AARP's income stream.

AARP received $838.7 million from "royalties:" payments received as a result of promotion of insurance and other products of value. AARP's magazine generated another $149.6 million from advertising, and AARP gained more than $91.4 million from grants, and another $93.1 million from fees paid to participate in its programs.

The AARP Foundation, according to auditors, received $78.7 million in federal government grants and another $542 million from various state programs.[2]

AARP has a vested interest in MediCratic health care. Each time a responsible member of Congress tries to advance Medicare reform, AARP notifies its members with strong messages of impending doom – fear is a strong motivator. The Congressman that truly wants to fix Medicare's

---
[1] "AARP Annual & Financial Reports- AARP, AARP Foundation and AARP Services Inc." AARP. Accessed May 16, 2017.
http://www.aarp.org/about-aarp/company/annual-reports/.
[2] Ibid.

$38 trillion unfunded liability with meaningful reforms will feel the wrath of the AARP members in his or her district. It is easy to be cynical about this: AARP seems interested in preserving its $1.5 billion empire, not preserving health care freedom for future generations.

AARP's reliance on non-membership income makes them operate more like an insurance marketing agency than an advocate for good public policy for seniors. Considering that voluntary membership dues are less than 19 percent of their income, many members likely join only to purchase the AARP endorsed insurance plans. Then, to add insult to injury, this billion dollar corporation's foundation receives more than $79 million in taxpayer funded grants. (Meanwhile, small business owners are struggling to keep their doors open, and one of the reason is they must pay taxes so that AARP and others can get grants.)

AARP endorsed the ACA, even though the new law promised to cut $700 billion from Medicare, and it continues to fight to keep the ACA in place. Does it strike you that perhaps AARP is more interested in insurance revenues from the sale of Medi-Gap policies than in representing the best interests of their members?

Representing physicians or themselves?

In a different chapter, we described the cozy relationship between the Centers for Medicare and Medicaid Services (CMS) and the American Medical Association (AMA). Even though the AMA represents only a small percentage of practicing physicians and surgeons, it has immense clout in Congress. The nearly $72 million in royalties from its CPT codes in 2010 is of more interest to the AMA than preserving health care freedom.23 In 2009, this CPT-code revenue was only $66 million, yet after the ACA passed, their revenues in 2010 rose to $72 million. Ironically, their income from CPT codes has started to fall as medical providers shift to ICD-10 coding. Does it strike you that the AMA's fervent support for the ACA stemmed more from increasing its CPT code revenue than from representing their members' best interests? Furthermore, does it strike you as odd that the AMA endorsed a plan based on cutting their members' reimbursements by 41 percent?

In 2015, the AMA strongly supported the Medicare Access and CHIP Reauthorization Act (MACRA). Ostensibly, this new law would free physicians from the threat of reimbursement cuts under the Sustained Growth Rate (SGR) plan. MACRA, however, still places physicians under the thumb of MediCrats at CMS and subject to their rate-setting. One would expect that an organization dedicated to bettering the professions of its members would advocate for more freedom, not less.

Of its $323.7 million 2016 income, only $39.1 million comes from membership dues[3] – 12 percent. It receives nearly as much – $39.1 million – from insurance commissions, and another $61.8 million from sales of books, newsletters, and other products. It held $510.8 million in permanent reserves and owns an insurance company.

As with many huge associations, the members often join because of the side benefits, not because the association represents their point of view. The AMA seems to bear witness to this irony, in that its membership appeals mostly to students, academic physicians and surgeons, and retired practitioners.

An indicator of AMA's political clout is found in President Obama's naming of Regina Benjamin, M.D., to be the 18th Surgeon General of the United States. Benjamin has a

---

[3] AMA Financial Statements. Report of the Board of Trustees, I-A-17. 2016.

long history of service to the American Medical Association. Her accomplishments can be lauded, but caused concern. Along with her AMA credentials, Benjamin has served on the boards of the Robert Wood Johnson Foundation, and Kaiser Commission on Medicaid and the Uninsured. Both of these groups have a well-earned reputation as favoring federal government programs. Certainly, the president has a right to appoint someone who believes as he does, and by her affiliations, Benjamin was a good choice for someone with Obama's point of view. However, her background did not give one much confidence that she believed in preserving a healthy free market for health care.

Big Pharma

Pharmaceutical companies have created medical miracles through prescription drugs. They have also created, through their advertising and sophisticated marketing systems, a national dependency on prescription medicines.

One can dispute the efficacy of this or that medicine. Indeed, some physicians almost refuse to prescribe prescription drugs, while others seem overly ready to do so. Yet, during the past 20 years prescription medicines have constituted 9.44 percent of our total spending on health care.[4] Obviously, Americans like what prescription medicines can do.

When it comes to reforming health care, the pharmaceutical companies jealously claimed their place at the table. They were not shy to elbow others aside to make sure that the MediCrats list their products as reimbursable under Medicare, Medicaid, and private insurance. Without convincing the MediCrats of the importance of their prescription drugs, the pharmaceutical companies would quit creating new medicines, or go out of business.

---

[4] CMS. *National Health Expenditures: Historical. 1960-2015.*

Rigged: How Insurance Ruined Health Care

During the debates about the Affordable Care Act of 2010, Big Pharma won a small, but important war against low cost alternatives. The ACA changed the rules about using Health Savings Accounts – along with HRAs and FSAs - to pay for over-the-counter medicine (OTC). Prior to the passage of the ACA, an individual could use their HSA/HRA/FSA to purchase lower cost OTC medicines. While the ACA law prohibits this, unless a physician writes a prescription, new Congressional reform efforts hopes to reinstate OTC medications as an eligible expense. This may seem small in terms of dollars, but it is a clear indicator of the power of the pharmaceutical companies to influence politicians.

Unions

During the congressional debate over the ACA, Democrats in Congress wanted to tax ultra-rich health care benefits – usually called Cadillac health plans. These health plans cover almost everything and feature co-pays as low as zero dollars to $5. Naturally, the monthly premiums are very high but they are fully tax-deductible to the employer, and not taxed to the employee.

With the Cadillac tax, Congress meant to tax benefits of rich executives. When the unions found out, however, they howled in protest. Many union health benefits far exceeded the $8,500 for an individual and $23,000 for a family – the original thresholds in the bill. Congress originally intended for these to take effect soon after it passed the ACA. Once the unions engaged however, Congress quickly backed off and settled on a Cadillac tax on health plans in excess of "…$10,200 for an individual or $27,500 for a family…The tax would not be imposed until 2018."[5] The ACA set the tax

---
[5] March 18, 2010. Retrieved on July 13, 2010.

rate at 40 percent of the premiums that exceed the threshold, a very high level of taxation. New reform efforts may not drop the Cadillac tax, but continue to push out its effective date – if it will ever happen.

Conservative commentators quickly picked up on the irony: Democrats in Congress meant to punish wealthy individuals, and found themselves punishing their rank and file union supporters. Congress quickly backed away. In fact, most commentators still believe the Cadillac tax will never go into effect, not because of wealthy individuals, but because the unions will never let it happen.

The health insurance companies

More than 1,300 health insurance companies are members of America's Health Insurance Plans (AHIP). AHIP's members provide health insurance coverage to more than 200 million Americans. In other words, AHIP is powerful.

AHIP, along with unions, AARP, Big Pharma, Kaiser, and major activist groups, had powerful influence on Congress when it wrote the ACA and continue to do so whenever health care reform emerges in Congress. There are very few institutions more hated than health insurance companies, and the companies know it, yet AHIP won a place at the table and fights to keep it, while negotiating with politicians and MediCrats.

AHIP is smart and wants to remain powerful. In July 2015, AHIP announced that it had secured Marilyn Tavenner as its new President. Tavenner promptly resigned her position as CEO of the Medicare system. From a principal regulator of insurance companies, Tavenner would join the fight

---

http://www.kaiserhealthnews.org/Stories/2010/March/18/Cadillac-Tax-Explainer-Update.aspx

with CMS and the federal government to advance AHIP's power to influence health insurance reform.

Politicians continually blast health insurance companies because the companies have the audacity to want to underwrite health risk. Underwriting is a method used by insurance companies to determine their financial risk and set premium rates. They do this by segregating individuals based on factors such as age, health, unhealthy practices, and geographic location. Underwriting makes insurance more affordable for healthy people, but that is not important to politicians. Politicians want to please as many voters as possible, especially those who have higher medical risks and are always vocal about it.

Insurance executives are at the mercy of Congress when they attempt to defend underwriting, especially when the Members just listened to a young mother whose baby died, an aging widow whose spouse died, or a disabled person sitting in the $30,000 wheelchair purchased by health insurance. AHIP clearly knew this battle had ended before it began. AHIP's primary concern is defending their members' interests, and the primary interest of health insurance companies is to make sure premium dollars fill their coffers.

AHIP decided soon after president Obama won election to make a deal with the MediCrats. If Congress agreed to include a legal requirement that everyone had to own health insurance, then the insurance companies would do away with underwriting. Anyone, regardless of health condition, would be able to purchase health insurance. Insurance premiums would be greatly equalized among healthy and unhealthy individuals.

AHIP had every reason to endorse guaranteed issue insurance without preexisting conditions. Why? If federal law forced everyone to own insurance, then healthy individuals who prefer not to own insurance would be required by law to purchase it. Healthy people would help underwrite the cost of unhealthy people, even though everyone would pay more. Health insurance companies understood this meant hundreds of billions of dollars in increased premium.

In June 2012, the Supreme Court ruled the ACA mandate to purchase insurance was a tax. It let the entire law bill stand as it regarded commercial and subsidized health plans. Health insurance companies hoped this would be enough to motivate people to buy health care before they get sick. For those that still refused to buy insurance there is a small IRS penalty to pay, one that is far less expensive than insurance. Because the law required insurance companies to issue coverage to anyone that wants to purchase it without any restrictions for medical conditions, and with the weak IRS tax penalty, insurance premiums have spiraled upward and have become unaffordable to millions of Americans. By 2017, several major insurance companies have quit selling individual health insurance policies, or at least, have quit offering coverage on government-run insurance exchanges. If the disastrous effects of ACA reforms are not corrected, It is likely that only a few, huge insurance companies will continue to stay in business, making health insurance unaffordable and very difficult to purchase.

The ACA and subsequent health insurance reforms rely on taxpayer subsidies to reduce an individual's net cost of insurance. AHIP couldn't be more pleased, even if most of the premium money comes from taxpayers – and the tax on insurance premiums. The billions in tax subsidies dos not come from thin air: it is money transferred from other sources using the power of the federal government to tax. Health insurance companies win – perhaps for a time – and taxpayers lose.

AHIP's power has allowed them to convince other health insurance professionals to support the individual mandate and tax-subsidized premiums. Major groups representing health insurance agents, third-party administrators, human resource professionals, and others jumped on board. The MediCrats won, and the people lost.

All thinking people realize that forcing individuals to purchase health insurance means health care spending will spiral upward. More individuals, physicians, hospitals, and other medical providers will become addicted to the increased cash raging like a wild river through the health care system.

Many health insurance agents believe they, too, benefit from the individual mandate, and the promise of more people buying health insurance. The ACA, however, also created the Medical Loss Ratio (MLR) formula that we wrote about in an earlier chapter. Suffice it to say, the MLR has already begun to reduce insurance agents' commissions to the point where some have quit, and many others will give up and find something else to do. Once again, the MediCrats will have won.

The MediCrats tipped their hand about health insurance agents in late 2008, in a study released by the Congressional Budget Office:

> In general, however, substantial reductions in administrative costs would probably require *the role of insurance agents and brokers in marketing and selling policies to be sharply curtailed and the services they provide to be rendered unnecessary.*[6] [Emphasis added.]

What difference does it make?

Under the new ACA rules negotiated by hundreds of

---

[6] Congressional Budget Office (2008, December). *Key Issues in Analyzing Major Health Insurance Proposals*. Washington, D.C., p. xv

Rigged: How Insurance Ruined Health Care

MediCrats, health care spending and insurance rates spiraled upward, along with taxes. One reason is that individuals are at the mercy of the health insurance exchanges and the rules MediCrats have designed to operate them. Without the help of a professional health insurance agent, and under the impression that more insurance is a better deal, health care spending has spiraled higher each year. In 2015, total health care spending totaled $3.2 Trillion, a 23 percent increase since 2010. From 17.3 percent of the United States Gross Domestic Product (GDP) in 2010, by 2015 health care spending consumed 17.7 percent of GDP – a significant increase in spending, given that the ACA's proponents promised a reduction in health care spending.[7]

Table 1 is included for illustration purposes, although the data dates to 2011. The type of HSA plan used in Table 1 is no longer available as a result of the ACA, but the idea the table demonstrates is still an important one. The premiums shown in Table 1 would likely be 200 percent or more greater using today's ACA-inflated rates.

Table 1 shows the foolishness of thinking a low co-pay is a good idea. Yet, the low co-pay is favored by the MediCrats, most of whom receive their insurance from a government agency.

Notice in the example that one column indicates a health plan with no office co-pay, while the other includes a $35 office co-pay. All other things being equal, the total potential out of pocket expense for a family under these two plans is $17,000 (an incredibly expensive burden on families). On the surface, it appears the $35 office co-pay is a better deal than the plan without an office co-pay where you may end up paying the full price of an office visit. Let's dig deeper.

---

[7] NHE, and https://www.statista.com/statistics/188105/annual-gdp-of-the-united-states-since-1990/

Rigged: How Insurance Ruined Health Care

	Table 1	
	Without Co-Pay	**With Co-Pay**
Single deductible	$ 2,500	$ 2,500
Family deductible	$ 5,000	$ 5,000
Co-Insurance	20%	20%
Out of Pocket	$ 3,000	$ 3,000
Family OOP	$12,000	$12,000
Office Co-Pay	--	35
Drug Co-Pay	0	15/35/65
Total OOP	$17,000	$17,000
Premium	$ 336.67	$ 641.57
Annual Premium	$4,040.04	$7,698.84
At risk before Co-Pay	$21,040.40	$24,698.84
Cost of Co-Pay Rider		$ 3,658.80
Monthly Cost of Co-Pay Rider		$ 304.90

Table 1 shows the total amount of insurance premium for these two plans. The plan without an office co-pay shows a annual premium of $4,040. The plan with an office co-pay shows a premium of $7,699. Adding the total potential out of pocket expenses for each plan we discover the cost of owning a $35 co-pay adds $3,659 to the richer health plan – $305 more a month.

You say, "Yes, but look at all I will save when I go to the doctor." Most people think that way, and it's why they pay far too much for health insurance. In a very bad year, a family may visit the doctor 20 times. If each of those visits cost the family $100, it equals $2,000 out-of-pocket for the year. If the family has a $35 office co-pay, instead of $2,000 the cost is only $700. It sounds on the surface as if the family saved $1,300. If, however, the added cost of the $35 co-pay's rider is added to the $700, the total rises to $4,358. This compares with $2,000 paid in cash, without the co-pay. Which of these two plans makes the most sense to you now?

There is more to this: When you pay an office co-pay, the insurance company never credits it against your deductible. If you pay without a co-pay, it is all credited against your deductible. Health insurance companies are not stupid. These health insurance plans are designed to take in more money than is spent – at least when all the premium of the company's insured people is added together.

You will always come out ahead owning a high deductible health plan without office co-pays if it is linked to other forms of health care consumerism, such as health insurance with a reference-based payment system and true pricing transparency (see Chapter 11).

One last note: HillaryCare and ObamaCare rested on different philosophical foundations

If the United States had a free market health care system, individual patients and their physicians would deal directly with each other on payment for care and decisions about which care is necessary. They would not first consult with the MediCrats or the MediCrats' book of rules.

In 1993, Hillary Rodham Clinton led an effort to reform the United States' health care system. The 1,368 page bill that resulted from her efforts – called HillaryCare – clearly rested on socialist economic models. Whether implicitly or explicitly, under HillaryCare the federal government controlled, or even owned, everything that mattered in the health care system. The federal government would have been in control.

> **SOCIALISM:** any of various economic and political theories advocating collective or governmental ownership and administration of the means of production and distribution of goods.[8]

Some individuals suggested that ObamaCare was a socialist system. It is not. ObamaCare relies on large organizations that can be controlled by MediCrats: health insurance exchanges, accountable care organizations, health insurance companies, pharmaceutical companies, all taking their orders from appointed federal government officials – this is the epitome of fascism.

> **FASCISM** : a political philosophy, movement, or regime (as that of the Fascisti) that exalts nation and often race above the individual and that stands for a centralized autocratic government headed by a dictatorial leader, severe economic and social regimentation, and forcible suppression of opposition.[9]

Why did Big Insurance oppose HillaryCare, but support ObamaCare? HillaryCare would have resulted in government ownership of health insurance: it would have rendered private health insurance to history's ash heap. ObamaCare, however, made no such assertion. Instead, it allowed private insurance – AHIP's members – to exist, although under strict federal control. The AHIP/MediCrat cabal resulted in an oligarchy of power common to fascism.

---

[8] Merriam Webster. (2011) Retrieved July 13, 2011. http://www.merriam-webster.com/dictionary/ socialism?show=0&t=1310584193

[9] Merriam Webster. (2011). Retrieved July 13, 2011. http://www.merriam-webster.com/dictionary/fascism

Rigged: How Insurance Ruined Health Care

It may seem reckless to use a term such as fascism to describe ObamaCare. It is not, because it is an accurate description of how it functioned. From the Independent Payment Advisory Board, comparative effectiveness studies, practice guidelines, CMS dictates, and the immense power vested in the Secretary of Health and Human Services, it is easy to see how ObamaCare fit the definition of fascism like a glove.

During the economic meltdown that started in 2007, we became used to the term "too big to fail." Pundits used this term to sell an idea. The idea they meant to sell was that huge banks and investment firms, General Motors, and Chrysler, are so important to our economy that if any of these were to go bankrupt, the economy would fail. ObamaCare comes at health care providers and payers in the same manner: The federal MediCrats will make sure that ACOs, exchanges, and all the other mega-players favored by politicians and special interest groups, will never fail – no matter what it costs everyday Americans.

One question that looms on the horizon: As with the financial collapse of 2008-2009, will ObamaCare have created a few "too big to fail" health insurance companies so that taxpayers will be hit up to bail them out? That question is being answered in states like Minnesota, which spent more than $300 million taxpayer dollars in 2017 to underwrite unaffordable insurance premiums for more than 100,000 individuals.

Chapter 5

Defeating Competition

Despite constant improvements in medical, surgical, pharmaceutical, and communication technology, health care spending, it seems, continues to spiral higher. Why? The opposite happened when technological research resulted in breakthroughs for consumer electronics.

Perhaps the classic story of how technology affects the price of something is the calculator. During the early 1960s, Texas Instruments came out with a hand sized electric calculator that sold for about $200 – equal to $1,608 in 2017. Today, you can purchase a notebook computer that not only has a calculator, but runs hundreds of software programs: It sells for less than $200.

When "car phones" first became available, heavy users spent more than $2,000 a month on usage charges. They paid huge extra charges for long distance calls, if they could even be made. Today, you can call toll free and purchase thousands of minutes at an affordable flat fee – and send photos of your favorite pet (or person) to your cousins in Madrid. In fact, long distance charges in the early 1970s were commonly $2 or more a minute (more than $11.45 today), but nearly every phone company offers free long distance today.

Thanks to advances in technology, computers, cell

phones, television sets, and a long list of other products and services sell for a fraction of their price just a few years ago. Why, then, is this not true with health care?

There are many instances where the price of medical care has gone down because of advances in technology. In the early 1990s when it was a new procedure, Lasik surgery cost $10,000 per eye. Today, Lasik surgeons advertise prices as low as $300 or $400. The average Lasik surgery today runs about $2,260 an eye (even in Canada).[1] Can you think of other medical procedures in which the cost has dropped 77 percent or more in the last 20 years?

In Milwaukee, Wisconsin, you can receive an MRI for $600 at Smart Choice MRI. The clinic offers a single flat price no matter what type of MRI your doctor orders. The clinic uses the most advanced technology to do its scans, and teleradiology to read them – all by radiologists at The Cleveland Clinic. At MediBid.com, you can find an even lower price for an MRI, often as low as $380.

Yet, unless you shop carefully, the price of your MRI might exceed $1,000, $2,500, $5,000 or more. There is a reason for this.

The sorry fact is that all medical procedures are price fixed. The CPT code system used to determine the reimbursement received by a physician or hospital makes no distinction within the same marketplace.

What do you call the person that finishes last in a medical school class?[2]

Consider Dr. Bright, who graduated first in his class at Harvard medical school, and Dr. Dull, who graduated last in his class from a third-rate medical school. Drs. Bright and

---

[1] https://www.qualsight.com/how-much-is-lasik
[2] Doctor.

Dull both practice at Big City Clinic. When Dr. Bright and Dr. Dull perform the same procedure, the Big City Clinic office clerk uses the same CPT code to bill it to the insurance company or patient. CPT codes do not discriminate based on quality of care or care-provider – only type of care provided.

Suppose that Dr. Bright can complete surgery in two hours. Dr. Dull performs the same procedure, but it takes him three hours. Since the CPT code is the same for the procedure, both doctors generate the same reimbursement for each procedure. Dr. Bright might earn more in fees, because he can do more procedures. Dr. Dull, on the other hand, might have to repeat some procedures, to get it right.

Dr. Bright and Dr. Dull know that patients seldom ask questions related to the price of health care. In fact, patients tend to ask only these two questions: Is it covered under my policy? Is Big City Clinic in my network?

The patient may never hear a physician ask this question, but the clerk at the registration desk most certainly will: "May I have your insurance card?" This is another way of saying, "Do you have health insurance, and if so, are we in your network?" The clerk has another reason, wanting to know how much the clinic will receive from the insurance company.

Neither the patient nor the physician talks about the price of care. The chances are that the physician has no clue about the price, and it is doubtful that anyone at Big City Clinic, save the business manager, knows the price of procedures. Dr. Bright and the patient are interested only in whether insurance pays for the procedure. If insurance does not pay, the chances are the procedure becomes "less necessary:" no wonder there is no competition in health care pricing.

As you can tell from the above and the previous chapters, the CPT code reimbursement system is based on price fixing, and it virtually prohibits competition in medicine.

Other People Pay and Process Claims

In Chapter 1 we saw that in 1919, insurance companies resisted writing health insurance policies because they understood how hard it would be to predict the use of health insurance. This is not to say that forms of insurance cannot be devised to pay for major medical and hospital claims. As a nation, we did that quite well up until 1965. Since it is impossible to accurately predict individual health care needs, we created a reimbursement system that pays medical providers after the fact. It relies on third-party payers – health insurance companies and the government – to reimburse physicians and hospitals, for routine and major medical expenses. As a result, we often spend health care dollars unnecessarily.

Our third-party payer system encourages wasteful spending. It nearly begs us is to use health insurance as much as we can so we feel that we get value for our premium dollars. This is worse under the new Medical Loss Ratio required by the ACA. During the four years immediately after Congress passed Medicare and Medicaid, annual health care spending spiraled upward at an average rate in excess of seven percent annually. Congress then created the Health Maintenance Organization (HMO) to extend comprehensive health benefits like those on Medicare and Medicaid enjoyed to people with private insurance. As a result, during the 10-year period from 1974 to 1983, annual health care spending increased an average of 15.8 percent per year.[3] When some-

---

[3] Table 12: *Per Enrollee Expenditures and Growth in medicare Spending and in Private Health Insurance premiums, Calendar Years 1969-2003*. Centers for Medicare and Medicaid Services. Washington, DC.

one else pays the bill – someone else being third-party payers – it provides incentive to spend more.

In an attempt to put the brakes on health care spending, Managed Care Organizations (MCO) became the rage. Neither HMOs nor MCOs, however, reduced total spending – the opposite happened. Why? Because patients no longer paid for their own care: third-party payers paid claims.

HMOs and MCOs severely damaged the physician-patient relationship. To control spending, HMOs, ACOs, and MCOs essentially provide incentives to physicians to deny care, especially when it relates to referrals to specialists.

Third-party payer schemes create other wasteful incentives. This happens when physicians are tempted to schedule patients for more than one appointment: if they can schedule a second appointment, they receive a second reimbursement..

> Although this happened in Canada, it can be repeated everywhere that physicians are paid based on a CPT-type reimbursement system. The patient (we will call her Terry) had terrible bunions on both feet. They hurt so bad that she had trouble walking.
>
> Terry went to Dr. Foote, her primary care physician and asked the doctor to look at her feet. She wanted relief – yesterday if possible. Dr. Foote looked at her right foot and declared, "Yes, this is serious. I will try to get you into an orthopedic surgeon."
>
> "Well, it's both feet," Terry told Dr. Foote.
>
> "I see," Foote replied. "Okay then, let's have you make an appointment at the next opening, and I will take a look at your left foot." You cannot make this stuff up: this actually happened – probably more often than known.

Dr. Foote knew the reimbursement rate for each clinic visit was $13.50. It took him only two minutes to look at Terry's foot and offer his profound diagnosis. No way did he want to keep the next patient waiting by looking at the left foot, too, especially when he would only receive $13.50 for the single visit.

Terry put her foot down (meaning, thereby, she screamed at Dr. Foote) and persuaded him to actually spend another two minutes with her. "Okay," he said, anxious to get to the next patient and another $13.50. "You need a bunionectomy. We'll get you into the queue. Last time I checked, it was about 32 months."

This true story ended well for Terry. She and her husband moved to the U.S.A. and she had surgery two days later at a cost of about $2,800.

With an HMO, or other managed care system, the incentive is to limit access to diagnostic tests and delay surgery. The patient is somewhat at the mercy of the MediCrats at Medicare, Medicaid, or the insurance company – the payers – unless their physician is aggressive and combative. If a third-party payer refuses to authorize you to see a specialist, your physician will have his or her hands tied. Instead of making a medical decision, your physician could be forced to make a reimbursement decision.

Let's face it: some patients are hypochondriacs and need to be told, "No." Some physicians have a hard time saying no. In these cases, the HMO can do some good, but at the cost of denying care to those who might really need it.

A better way to skin the dollars

There is a far better way to decide when to spend health care dollars than be at the mercy of a third-party payer: The best way to do this is for the patient, you, to have "skin in the game." In other words, the patient should be responsible for a portion of his or her medical and hospital expense. The portion can vary, but the greater it is, the more careful the patient becomes about how to spend health care dollars.

Consider Joe Smith. Joe's employer provides him and his family with a health insurance plan. Joe pays $300 a month to cover his family, and $200 a month to cover himself – Joe's employer pays the balance of $1,600. Joe's insurance policy has a $500 deductible, and 100 percent coverage for preventive care. To make it even "better" for Joe, his employer will reimburse the $500 Joe might spend on health care. In other words, the health care that Joe uses will cost him nothing out of his pocket. It's expensive, however, and Joe feels cheated if he doesn't use it – often.

Joe's daughter twisted her ankle while playing soccer. Joe left the soccer field and took her directly to the emergency room. He demanded she receive not only an x-ray, but an MRI. The E.R. physician told Joe the x-ray was conclusive: There was no damage to his daughter's ankle. Still, Joe pushed the E.R. doctor for the MRI. The doctor had to call the insurance company to receive permission, and it was denied. This meant telling Joe "no" once again. Joe had no idea that this emergency room visit cost in excess of $2,500, and that the hospital would have added $3,200 more just for the MRI. Why? He paid nothing out of his pocket, and neither did he think twice of using the emergency room.

The next day, Joe's daughter's ankle hurt, and she limped slightly. Otherwise, she felt fine. "Coach says I should be able to play in two or three days," she told her dad.

Rigged: How Insurance Ruined Health Care
Jane Smith, Joe's sister-in-law

Now consider Jane Smith, Joe's sister-in-law. Jane is self-employed and pays for health insurance for the Smith family. Sure enough, Jane can deduct 100 percent of her premium from her business income, thereby reducing her taxes. By 2016, thanks to the ACA, however, her family health plan cost had soared to $1,800 to pay the premium for her family. Jane tired of paying so much for insurance, and believed it was smarter to save money.

Jane's health insurance agent helped her find a high deductible health plan, with a $5,950 deductible for her family. Her premium fell to $485 a month, instead of $1,300 a month. Jane saved almost $10,000 a year by choosing the $6,000 deductible insurance plan.

Jane's son jammed his finger playing baseball. He demanded that Jane take him to the emergency room immediately. "Well, can you move the finger?" Jane asked.

"Yes, but it hurts real bad," her son said.

"Let's go home and put some ice on it. We'll see how it looks in the morning." Jane loved her son as much as Joe loved his daughter. Jane knew, however, she would have had to pay out of her own pocket (or her HSA) if she took her son to the emergency room. Without a doubt, she would have used the E.R. if she believed it was an emergency. Common sense told her otherwise.

The next day, Jane's son had a sore finger, but it was already on the mend. "Coach said I should be able to play in two or three days," he told his mother.

Jane and Joe dealt with similar injuries in completely different ways, based on who paid the bill. Neither child suffered needlessly, and each received necessary medical care. Joe spent $2,500 out of someone else's pocket, and Jane saved $2,500 out of her own pocket. This is what happens when individuals have "skin in the game."

If patients had more skin in the game they would more carefully make the decision when to purchase health care. Patients, along with their physicians, would decide whether to spend money on a specialist. The common option, unfortunately, is the one that is becoming more unaffordable every day. When a government bureaucrat or liberal activist says people cannot afford health insurance, or are underinsured, what they mean is that low deductible health insurance – the kind Joe Smith has – is too expensive. Jane may not like paying $485 a month for high deductible insurance, but it is more affordable than what Joe's employer pays – and Jane has the security of knowing major medical and hospital bills will be paid so the family can avoid bankruptcy. Always remember, the true purpose of insurance is to protect assets, not to pay for routine care.

Why not use cheaper help?

There are some who think that if clinics used physicians' assistants (PA), or nurse practitioners (NP), instead of medical doctors, the price of health care could be reduced. Experience is showing otherwise. Missouri added a new type of medical professional to meets its citizens' need for more doctors – Assistant Physicians.A controversial new law in Missouri will allow medical school graduates who haven't yet passed their final credentialing exam to treat patients in underserved primary care settings. …

… the law creates the new position of "assistant physician." These doctors would be supervised on site by a collaborative physician for 30 days. After that, they could treat patients without direct supervision in settings 50 miles away and will be able to prescribe Schedule III, IV, and V drugs.[4]

Because APs, PAs and NPs lack the medical knowledge, skills, and experience of a medical doctor, they tend to order more expensive and a greater number of diagnostic tests. The savings in the family practice clinic are lost in the MRI or specialist clinic. It might be that the family practice clinic earns as much, or even more money by using APs, and PAs, but the insurance company will pay out more because of the added diagnostic tests.

Why would you be willing to pay a Nurse Practitioner, a Physicians' Assistant, or an almost-a-doctor Assistant Physician the same high fees as you would to a medical doctor?

> Rudy and his wife Terry* went together to see a dermatologist. Instead of a medical doctor, a nurse practitioner treated them. The care they received was adequate, but they were outraged when they saw the final bill.
>
> The dermatology clinic had billed Rudy and Terry at the same rate as if they had seen the medical doctor. Terry called the health insurance company to complain. "We don't really care," the health insurance MediCrat responded.
>
> Because Rudy and Terry have skin in the game (a high deductible health plan and an HSA) they demanded an adjustment. If their insurance paid for the service, they would have ignored the price, although they might have still grumbled about the insurance company's indifference.

---

[4] Crane, Mark. "Missouri Law Creates New 'Assistant Physician' Designation." Medscape, July 15, 2015.
http://www.medscape.com/viewarticle/828255.

Why should insurance companies care if a clinic bills the same charge for an AP, PA, NP, and MD? Insurance companies have a vested interest in paying a large number of claims. The more claims they pay, the more premium they can collect. They earn their income based on how much premium they can collect, and how efficiently they can manage and invest the premium.

There is confusion about how medical clinics bill for the services of a non-physician as opposed to an MD. In some cases and under some conditions the clinic is reimbursed at the same rate no matter if a physician or a physician's assistant provides the care. In other cases, the clinic codes differently for the PA and the MD. The rules are complex. Much of it depends on how a billing clerk enters the CPT codes, and it is not hard to imagine that this creates an incentive for a clinic to use less skilled medical providers, and charge the same as they would for a professional physician.

Oftentimes, a surgeon has an attending physician by his or her side during a procedure. The lead surgeon receives 100 percent of the reimbursement rate for his or her services. The attending physician receives a percentage of the lead surgeon's fee. If, however, the attending medical professional is a PA instead of an MD, the reimbursement rate might be the same. In other words, either you are overpaying the physician's assistant, or underpaying the assisting medical doctor.

To Save Money: Buying Insurance Across State Lines

One very popular idea to reduce the cost of health insurance is to allow people to buy across state lines. For instance, a person living in Illinois could be given the option to buy insurance from a Colorado company. A Michigander should be able to buy insurance from an Arizona insurance company. The decision should be up to the individual, not to state or federal regulators. Perhaps the individual would find that even a smaller insurance company in a different state would offer more services at less cost.

There are several advantages to this idea of buying health insurance across state lines, but there are some serious problems.

Each state levies taxes on health insurance, and the taxes vary from state to state. If you could purchase insurance in a low tax state, the premium should be less. In a high tax state, all other things being equal, the premium would cost more.

There could be some administrative efficiencies resulting in savings for insurance companies that can sell in several states. A larger insurance company might be able to negotiate better reimbursement rates with physicians and hospitals than a small, regional or state insurance company. Then again, a smaller company may provide better customer service.

The number of mandates on insurance makes a huge difference. We covered this in Chapter 3. Some states require insurance policies to cover dozens of procedures, while other states only require a small number.

Relying on provider networks makes it more difficult to get real competitive prices. Suppose you own an Idaho policy, but you live in Ohio. It is very possible that your Idaho policy will not cover medical services provided by Ohio networks, simply because the Idaho insurance company does not have a provider network contract in Ohio. Idaho might reimburse at an "out of network" rate, and it usually means paying less of your medical bill to a physician – and you pay more.

Rigged: How Insurance Ruined Health Care

Medical providers often have network contracts with dozens of different health plans. This is very cumbersome and expensive. As a result, medical providers tend to resist signing new health plan contracts. This limits competition between medical providers and insurance companies. If an Ohio medical clinic signed new contracts with the Idaho insurance company, the reimbursement rates would be similar to those offered by an Ohio insurance company. It is hard to imagine medical clinics trying to manage contracts with insurance companies from 50 different states, and it is why providers resist signing new contracts.

It is just as likely that for an Idaho insurance company to be able to sell in Ohio, it must also cover all the same mandates. Ohio has 29 mandates while Idaho has 13: it is likely that an Idaho policy issued for someone who lives in Ohio would also cost more for the Ohioan. One way to deal with this is to have the federal government set the guidelines for all insurance policies, across all state lines but this would be terrible mistake. In fact, that is one of the things the ACA attempts to do – and the people in Idaho and Ohio will be penalized, as the number of mandates increases. Letting the federal government decide assumes Washington, D.C. MediCrats know more than the lawmakers in Ohio and Idaho – or wherever you live. Idahoans are by nature people of liberty, and are in for a rude awakening when federal government MediCrats tell them they must increase their mandates by 300-500 percent.

Having 50 state departments of insurance does create a lot of redundancies, overlap and waste. At the same time, letting the federal government regulate state health insurance creates a field ripe for the dictates of D.C. MediCrats.

The idea of selling health insurance across state lines is a good one. What complicates it so much, is our reliance

85

on a third-party payer system. All of the complications mentioned above are related to the fact that we expect health insurance to pay for just about everything, so we won't personally have to pay for very much.

How about allowing doctors to compete across state lines?

A better idea to reduce the price of health care is to allow doctors to compete across state lines for the same patients. If you live in Memphis, Tennessee, perhaps you want to go to Northeast Mississippi to save money on a medical procedure. If you live in St Paul, Minnesota, you might want to go to Hudson, Wisconsin, to save money on a medical procedure. It is unlikely, under today's rules that this will happen very often.

Physicians need credentials to be considered legitimate practitioners. This includes things like a medical license and board certification in their specialty. The requirements for credentials vary from state to state.

Each state has a medical board that determines the requirements for practice within its boundaries. A Mississippi physician might have different requirements imposed on him or her than a Tennessee counterpart. The state medical boards that determine credentials tend to strongly resist physicians crossing state lines to practice, and that is where medical politics can restrict the supply of physicians.

However, if the Memphis doctor is visited by a Mississippian, then the Tennessee rules apply. One very good reason for crossing state lines is that a certain procedure might be allowed in a doctor's clinic in one state, while it requires hospitalization in another.

These types of rules greatly increase the cost discrepancies between one state and another. As a result, buying an insurance policy from a low-cost state and using it in a high cost state may not be as effective as people believe.

Medical facilities – hospitals, clinics, urgent care centers, outpatient surgical centers, etc. – grant differing practice privileges to physicians based on a variety of criteria. If Dr. Foote wants to do bunionectomies at Big City Hospital, he must meet the criteria set by the hospital. The hospital relies on the Joint Commission (JCAHO) to determine most of its rules, but a hospital peer group (doctors) can help to control who receives privileges and who does not.

One reason your family practice doctor cannot perform certain procedures in his or her clinic is because of JCAHO rules. The JCAHO sets guidelines about where procedures will be performed. Who is the Joint Commission?

> The Joint Commission accredits and certifies more than 19,000 health care organizations and programs in the United States. Joint Commission accreditation and certification is recognized nationwide as a symbol of quality that reflects an organization's commitment to meeting certain performance standards.[5]

Third-party payers, whether private insurance companies or government health plans, will only pay if a facility has met JCAHO and board certified standards.

So whether directly or indirectly, state medical boards and hospital peer groups can have a limiting effect on the doctors that practice within each state. Unfortunately, the combination of state medical boards, facility peer groups, and JCAHO certification, limits the ability of physicians to compete across state lines. Ultimately, the individual chooses whether to travel to a different state to see a doctor. The doctor's license and any restrictions it applies are unrelated to

---

[5] *About the Joint Commission.* Retrieved July 8, 2011. http://www.jointcommission.org/about_us/about_the_joint_commission_main.aspx

the patient's residence. This provides at least some level of consumer choice, and could save patients money.

MediCrats Have Muddied the Competitive Waters

When the AMA, CMS, medical boards, JCAHO, insurance companies, and a host of other alphabet agencies combine their influence and resources, it inhibits price competition among medical providers. The MediCrats – the bureaucrats who control medical care supply and pricing – fight to retain their influence at every level.

> Sally Jones is a nervous woman. She has trouble sleeping, and is easily irritated. Sally went to her family physician, Dr. Calm, seeking relief. Dr. Calm talked with Sally for two minutes. Then the doctor opened a desk drawer, pulled out a questionnaire, and set it in front of Sally. "Take a few minutes with this and answer the questions," Dr. Calm said. "I will be right back," he said, leaving the PHQ-9 form for her to complete.
>
> When Dr. Calm returned, he saw that Sally's score on the questionnaire exceeded 12, indicating she may suffer mild depression. Based on this questionnaire, designed by MediCrats, Dr. Calm recommends that Sally should start taking Prozac.
>
> It took two years before Sally decided she had had enough. She demanded that Dr. Calm take her off Prozac. She hated the side effects.
>
> Dr. Calm recommended that Sally should see a psychiatrist or psychologist. Sally spent one day a week the next ten weeks talking with Ms. Mind, a psychol-

ogist. Ms. Mind showed Sally ways to relax and to confront the anger that resulted in "depression" – Ms. Mind called it "mild emotional discomfort."

"Why didn't they send me to you right away?" Sally asked.

"Well, Dr. Calm followed the practice guidelines, based on the score on your PHQ-9 questionnaire." MediCrats, including federal and state government regulators, third-party payers, peer groups, JCAHO, and medical boards all played a role in developing this protocol. Dr. Calm treated Sally correctly, based on the MediCratic guidelines.

MediCrats treat patients as if they were all the same. They are bean counters, and so, rely on ever-growing databases to determine which procedures they approve, and which they will reimburse. The statistics showed that for individuals with a score greater than 10 on the PHQ-9 questionnaire used by Dr. Calm, the recommended procedure was prescribing anti-depressants. Statistics showed Prozac worked with a large number of patients. That is why Sally's insurance company would pay for the prescription, but not for the services of a psychologist.

It is hard to blame physicians for this MediCratic system of health care delivery. Today's medical schools train them this way, and very few physicians deal with billing for medical services or collecting the bills. Physicians also know that following MediCratic guidelines is good defensive medicine that may reduce the threat of lawsuits.

MediCrats are primarily interested in determining the least costly way of delivering health care. Their best offensive weapon is to limit medical reimbursements, and eliminate real price competition.

Another hindrance to the power of competition

Most locales use "Certificate of Need Laws" to control the number of medical facilities in a location. The MediCrats believe that with these laws they can pre-determine how much capacity any area needs to meet the needs of its residents. This is yet another way to stifle competition.

In Tennessee, if an entity wishes to explore building a hospital, it must pay a $20,000 non-refundable fee to receive a permit. After paying the fee, however, MediCrats may deny the hospital's request, and refuse to issue a permit. Other medical facilities that do not want new competition can influence this permitting process through local politics and other forms of persuasion.

With other types of businesses, the market sorts this out, by rewarding the best businesses with more clients and by forcing other businesses to either improve, reduce prices, or quit. In the United States' health care system, Certificate of Need Laws reduce competition, increase prices, and force patients to flee the state, or the country for medical care.

Chapter 6:

Chargemaster Charade

Everyone knows Wal-Mart advertises that it discounts the price of everything it sells. When Wal-Mart says it is selling a $1,000 TV for $695, we all understand the real price is $695. Most likely, $695 is the price a person would always pay for that TV at Wal-Mart, until the merchandise became very old and hard to sell. Everyone that buys that specific Wal-Mart TV will pay the same price.

At a Target Super Store, if the label on a package of hamburger says $3.59 a pound that is the base price. If you buy two pounds, you will pay $7.18 – three pounds will be $10.77. The person standing behind you and in front of you will pay the same rate - $3.59 a pound. Everyone that buys hamburger on the same day pays the same.

When you walk into Macy's to buy a shirt you look at the price tag: $85. If you buy the red shirt and the man behind you buys the same shirt, but in blue, you will both pay $85. Macy's has sales from time to time and might discount the shirt to $69. The price, however, is transparent to everyone, where you can see it. Everyone that buys the shirt that same day pays $69.

Whether at Wal-Mart, Target, or Macy's, everyone pays the same price for the same object purchased on the same day. Employees may have a discount card, but all employees get the same discount or the shopper might have a coupon, but everyone with the same coupon pays the same price. The price is right on the label where you can see it. You pick it up, inspect it, furrow your brow, think about how much money is in your checkbook or available on a credit or debit card, and decide whether to make a purchase.

We are used to buying products and services at a price that is both transparent and predictable. We assume that everyone pays the same price. When it comes to health care, this is not true.

Health care providers hide the real price of medical care. They use a chargemaster pricing system that obscures the price, and results in dozens of different prices for the same service on the same day. "Patients pay as much as 683% more for the same medical procedures, such as MRIs or CT scans, in the same town, depending on which doctor they choose..."[1]

In a story following in a few pages, you will see how the chargemaster price actually was 2,000 percent greater than the cash price. Almost no one pays the "retail price" – the chargemaster price – for medical care. Instead, our MediCratic health care system puts patients at the mercy of a complex, opaque, unfair, and confusing billing process.

Years ago, when someone bought a new or used car, they ignored the sticker price – the dealer pasted it on a window so anyone could see it. Despite the sticker price, we knew the real price came after negotiating a discount directly with the salesman, the sales manager, and the finance department. The sticker price is like the health care chargemaster price, and the price one actually paid for the car is more like the provider network discounted price. Hey, maybe used

---

[1] Kennedy, K. (2011). "Health care costs vary widely, study shows." *USA Today*. Retrieved on July 19, 2011.
http://www.usatoday.com/cleanprint/?unique=1311082903145.

car salesman invented the chargemaster price!

The health care chargemaster price is usually as much as 200-600 percent -- sometimes even 2,000 percent -- higher than most people will actually pay. The difference in what a person pays is based on whether he or she has health insurance, with whom, and under whichever plan they are covered. How much the plan is paying to access the PPO network or HMO also adds to the price.

In truth, however, most people have no clue the price they are really paying because it is actually paid by a third party on their behalf. Insurance companies and government health plans negotiate discounts from the chargemaster price. If there is something akin to the real price of a health care service, it may be defined as whatever is closest to the average paid on behalf of everyone.

It is not a stretch to say that the chargemaster price is a phony price. Here are some clarifying examples:

Four Patients and a CEO

Amir Habib,[2] a multimillionaire Yemeni businessman, flew to Wheeling, West Virginia to visit the Wheeling Cardio Clinic. Habib had been suffering from sharp, stabbing pains in his chest. His personal physician suggested that he undergo a thorough cardiovascular evaluation. Hence, his trip to West Virginia, where he can be sure of getting high quality medical care.

Although money was no object, Habib was no fool. He negotiated a discounted price with the Cardio Clinic before flying to America. The clinic's business office told Habib that the total price of this thorough, sophisticated exam was $20,000. If, however, Habib paid in cash, they would discount it $5,000 – he would pay $15,000. Habib

---

[2] Ficticious name.

smiled and had his aide pay the bill immediately upon checking in at the clinic.

Perry Harte[3] also suffered chest pains. His family practice physician suggested he undergo a thorough examination at the Wheeling Cardio Clinic. Harte paid his $150 hospital admission co-pay upon checking in, and underwent the procedure. Forty-five days later, Harte received an Explanation Of Benefits (EOB) letter from his insurance company.

The EOB stated that the price for the procedure was $20,000, just as the clinic had quoted Habib. According to the EOB, Harte's insurance company showed Wheeling Cardio Clinic's responsibility was $12,000 – Harte's share was $8,000. Harte smiled, feeling grateful for the incredible discount negotiated by his insurance company. At the bottom of his bill, it said: "Your Share – $500." Harte's employer provided $500 deductible insurance, and he promptly sent a check to the clinic, covering his deductible. The insurance company paid $7,500.

Pete Elder[4] showed his Medicare card to the admitting clerk at Wheeling Cardio Clinic. Ninety days after having his cardiovascular evaluation, Elder received an EOB from Medicare, and another one from his AARP supplemental insurance company. He paid very little attention to either of the EOBs, only checking to make sure he owed nothing. Elder, had he studied the EOB, would have learned that Medicare authorized $3,500 for the test. Medicare paid $2,800, and Elder's AARP supplemental policy paid the rest.

Mary Paine[5] walked into the Wheeling Cardio Clinic. "I'm having these sharp stabbing pains in my chest," she told the triage nurse. Wheeling Cardio Clinic admitted her, despite the fact that she had no health insurance. Luckily for

---

[3] Ficticious name.
[4] Ficticious name.
[5] Ficticious name.

Mary, her condition could be treated with simple aspirin and a beta blocker. Her financial condition, however, had no treatment. The clinic billed Paine $20,000 for the evaluation. Paine paid as much as she could; about $20 a month – $750 over three years. Then she quit paying. The clinic went after her, but she filed bankruptcy.

During the next West Virginia legislative session, Fred Counter,[6] the CEO at Wheeling Cardio Clinic, testified before the Commerce Committee. Counter meant to persuade the legislators to appropriate more money for Medicaid patients, and create a fund for people like Mary Paine. "Times are tough at the clinic," Counter said. "Last year, just on our cardiovascular evaluation program alone, we lost $1.5 million. This resulted from people going without insurance and being unable to pay their bills."

"Mr. Counter," asked Senator Smart,[7] "when you say you lost $1.5 million, what do you base that on?" Senator Smart knew about the chargemaster billing system. He knew the average reimbursement received by Wheeling Cardio Clinic for the cardiovascular evaluation program was closer to $7,000, not the $20,000 Mr. Counter used to claim the clinic had lost so much money.

Wheeling Cardio Clinic's Contracts

Wheeling Cardio Clinic is reimbursed for services in number of different ways. It has contracts with insurance companies. It accepts payment from Medicare, Medicaid, Tricare, and other government health plans. There are also the cash customers. The MediCrats for each of these health plans negotiates with the MediCrats at Wheeling Cardio

---

[6] Ficticious name.
[7] Ficticious name.

Rigged: How Insurance Ruined Health Care

Clinic to agree on a reimbursement price for clinical services, making sure the respective MediCrats are satisfied.

It is common for a medical provider to receive reimbursements at dozens of different prices for the same service from the same payer, even when services are performed on the same day in the same location. Healthy Lives insurance Company (HLIC) may have five, 10, 15, or more contracts with Wheeling Cardio Clinic, each of which pays a different rate for the same procedure. HLIC will have one contract for West Virginia State employees, one for Wheeling city employees, a different one for county and school district employees (where it offers separate plans to professional and non-professional staff), another for Black Dust Coal Miners, three plans for Large Things Manufacturers, five different plans for small business owners, and nine different plans for individuals. Each plan negotiates its own contracted price with Wheeling Cardio Clinic.

No matter the negotiated price, Wheeling Clinic will always bill out $20,000 for the procedure. HLIC may pay $6,250 for the exam when given to state employees. It may pay $7,000 for employees of the Black Dust Coal Mining. For individual insurance and small business plans, it might pay $9,750. Remember, these are payments for the identical service performed on the same date in the same location.

Carol Common[8] has her health insurance with Oldtimers Fraternal, and is covered under an indemnity plan. Oldtimers does not have a contract with Wheeling Cardio Clinic, but the insurance pays 80 percent of the clinic's usual and customary charge. Oldtimers pays Wheeling Cardio Clinic 80 percent of $20,000 – $16,000.

(Stop for a moment now and think about buying a shirt at Macy's based on your Clothing Network Card. You are standing at the checkout counter watching 27 other people

---

[8] Ficticious name.

buy the same shirt on the same day. The cash register shows the price each pays for the "$85" shirt: $42.65, $78, $67.22, $39.87 ["Whew," you say, wondering what kind of network to which that man belongs], and so forth. The man in front of you pays $85, apparently not noticing or caring what others paid. You hold your breath – $54.16. Okay, you can go with it. Now you know why the MediCrats do all they can to avoid transparency.)

The actual average reimbursement for the cardiovascular exam in our example is $7,000. Why, then, doesn't Wheeling Cardio Clinic settle on the same price for everyone?

Proving their worth?

When Wheeling Cardio Clinic patients receive an EOB in the mail, they like to see the discount. It gives them confidence that their insurance company is working hard on their behalf to hold health care prices down. The chargemaster system, then, provides a marketing advantage for insurance companies. It makes them appear to be more valuable than they really are.

True enough, the mega insurance companies can apply maximum leverage to smaller medical clinics to win lower contract prices. On the other hand, mega medical clinics can apply maximum leverage on insurance companies to win higher contracted prices. That is one reason why in the same city or town, physicians, surgeons, hospitals, medical clinics, and other medical providers, are paid at different rates – it is a primary reason why it is nearly impossible for you to know the price of medical and hospital care.

Rigged: How Insurance Ruined Health Care
A critical problem

The chargemaster price is used to allow medical providers to collect more from cash paying patients and indemnity companies. It is also applied when an individual receives care but is insured by a company with whom the provider has no contract. Read the following description of an actual case from Florida:

> There was a dispute between BayCare Health System Inc. of South Florida and an insurance network called Health Options. A pricing agreement between the two parties had been allowed to lapse after the two failed to agree on what constituted reasonable prices. So the hospital, no longer bound by a contract, chose to bill the insurance network the full chargemaster prices (and expect payment in full).

> The Florida legislature had put in place an independent tribunal to settle such disputes between insurance plans and hospitals. The two disputants took the matter to this independent tribunal, and the tribunal determined for them what constituted the right price: Medicare plus 20%.

> An excerpt from a newspaper column discussing the case follows:

> Florida's largest health insurance company scored a huge victory over a billing dispute with Tampa Bay's area's main hospital group.

> In its claims dispute, BayCare argued that since there was no contract in effect, Health Options is required to pay what was billed and that those charges were, in fact, "usual and customary charges."

However, state records indicate that BayCare didn't "provide the rationale for its assertion." Health Options reimbursed the facilities at 120 percent of the Medicare participating rate and provided a "detailed" reason why the level was usual and customary, state records show. The difference between what BayCare billed for emergency services and what Health Options reimbursed is about $1.45 million."[9]

It's not just insurance companies that get overcharged by the chargemaster system, as BayCare did in Florida. The Rooney-Perrin book from which the story came also describes everyday citizens who, upon receiving their hospital bills, discovered they, too, had been billed the chargemaster price. Since these overcharged patients had no idea what the real average price of care was, they felt obligated to pay the chargemaster price – or perhaps went bankrupt instead. Using the BayCare case as a precedent, individuals find they can fight the medical provider and win a huge discount. Perhaps, if they are tough enough, they can pay no more than Medicare plus 20 percent.

Only uninformed, uneducated individuals – or fools – pay the full chargemaster price.

Exaggerated discounts on medical tourism

We cover medical tourism in a different chapter, but these comments relate to the chargemaster price system.

Surprisingly, when you need a surgical procedure, a medical tourism broker can show you how to save 40 percent, 50 percent, or even 75 percent by traveling to a foreign country to receive care. To make these discounts seem so

---

[9] Rooney, P.; Perrin, D. (2208). *America's health care Crisis Solved. Money-saving Solutions, Coverage for Everyone.* John Wiley & sons, Inc, Hoboken, New Jersey. P 90-91.

large, the broker shows you the U.S. chargemaster price, not the average reimbursed price. Comparing charges for surgery in a foreign country with the chargemaster price at a U.S. hospital is as different as comparing the prices of filet mignon and Spam.

The chargemaster price for a knee replacement in a major metropolitan area of the United States could be $60,000. The average price actually paid by insurance companies might be $25,000 to $30,000. The medical tourist broker will show how an individual can receive the same service in India, Thailand, or Costa Rica for $15,000. The broker brags that he or she has saved the patient $45,000, but the broker does not mention he or she is paying the medical provider only $10,000.

You may have been able to find a willing medical provider in the United States that would accept $15,000 to $20,000 for the same service. If you are willing to travel, the cost may be as low as $7,500. Go to MediBid.com – and it may not require you to travel internationally. MediBid.com's price is based on what a willing provider would charge, not on a phony comparison with the chargemaster price.

Chargemaster price is opaque insurance companies and providers like it that way

Health care payers and providers in the United States have found a way to keep milking the cash cow. All they must do is hide the real price of health care by using the chargemaster billing system, and low-deductible, low co-pay prepaid health plans. If your employer or you are willing to pay ever-increasing insurance premiums, and not worry about the real price of care, this system will continue to operate. Your cost will continue to go up every year.

There really is no incentive for health insurance companies and medical providers to tell you the real price of care; that is, unless you own a high deductible insurance policy and pay the first dollars of your care out of your own pocket. Then, price transparency is extremely important – so is paying the lowest possible price.

This is a true story, although the name was changed. Terry needed surgery.

> Terry and her husband consulted with a hospital that expected to be paid $22,000 for the procedure. Terry owned a high deductible health insurance plan. She knew that the couple would have to pay around the first $7,000 out of their own pocket. Their insurance carrier either could not or would not provide them with an accurate estimate.
>
> The couple negotiated with a hospital until they found a price they were willing to pay: $1,300.

Try it, you might find it works for you. Or try MediBid.com where physicians and surgeons will deal directly with you.

Those of us who are not MediCrats, and are tired of paying overly expensive insurance premiums, have a vested interest in demanding an honest health care pricing system. An honest pricing system would be transparent. We would always know the average price paid by everyone for the same service, on the same day, at the same location. If Wal-Mart, Target, and Macy's can do it, so can medical providers like Wheeling Cardio Clinic and BayCare Hospital.

Rigged: How Insurance Ruined Health Care

CHAPTER 7

HOW PPOS PREVENT TRANSPARENCY AND INCREASE YOUR COSTS

"How much does it cost?" is a common question when we buy something. When it comes to health care the answer is three-fold: 1) it depends on your provider network, 2) it's purposely complex, and 3) it depends on which doctor you see.

Congress passed the Health Maintenance Organization (HMO) Act in 1973 in response to a rapid increase in health care spending triggered by the launch of Medicare and Medicaid in 1966. HMOs immediately proved popular and the insurance industry needed a competitive answer. The insurance industry responded to this HMO competition with a new idea: the PPO.

PPO means Preferred Provider Organization. The PPO is a network of medical doctors, hospitals, and other health care providers. PPOs remain the most common form of non-HMO health plans today.

Insurance companies claimed that PPOs would reduce the cost of health care services (how is that working out?). The reduction was to result from the insurance company contracting with the medical providers for a set price per service (or device, etc.). The insurance company claimed to be discounting the medical provider's price.

When we think of a discounted price, perhaps a one-day sale at a reputable department store comes to mind. In the previous chapter we talked about a shirt that sells every day for $85. Sometimes, however, the store discounts the shirt at a one-day sale price for, say, $59.99. Health care discounts, however, work differently.

Of course, some stores have huge sales on "Black Friday" or Christmas "sales." The discounts look great, but in fact, stores may mark up the price just days before the sale to make it look more like a steal of a deal.

Think of health care pricing more like buying a box spring and mattress. On the bed you see a label that says $1,295 – the List Price. Then you see the "Sale" tag pinned to the List Price, and it says $775 – the price you will pay. The fact is no one pays $775 – the List Price, and everyone gets a "Sale" price – the discount. Or do they?

When you "purchase" medical services or devices, the medical provider seldom shows or tells you a price. Instead, the provider sends a bill to the insurance company and the bill indicates the List Price – the Chargemaster Price. You read about this in Chapter 6.

The Chargemaster Price for a service might be $1,295. No one pays $1,295, however, except some few uninsured people who don't know better. Everyone in a PPO network gets a "discount" – the negotiated price paid to the PPO network providers.

Health insurance companies market their products in part by featuring their "discounts." By this they imply they offer the deepest discount, or the most affordable insurance option.

After you have "consumed" a service that is covered by your insurance plan, you eventually receive an EOB –

Explanation of Benefits – in the mail. It shows you the chargemaster price – the price no one pays – and the price your insurance will pay. The $1,295 "List Price" will be reduced to something more like $727.53. This price is usually called the "allowable" price. You smile because you escaped paying the high price. The EOB also shows you the portion you pay directly, the deductible, co-pay or co-insurance – perhaps $65. This all sounds like a great deal – but the discount is greatly exaggerated.

Re-Pricing

As a result of the chargemaster pricing system, a new industry has sprung up – "repricers." The repricer is another type of MediCrat. The repricer plays on people's ignorance of medical care pricing and the fear that comes when they see a huge bill they cannot pay.

The repricer appears after an uninsured person, or someone with a very high deductible health plan, has already received medical care. Repricers offer to "negotiate" a discounted price for the beleaguered debtor. The discounted price is calculated off the chargemaster price, but can be a great deal more than the price paid by a PPO. The repricer earns a percentage fee for all the money he or she has "saved" the debtor.

Sometimes repricers will buy the hospital's debt at a discount. The hospital is happy, because they have received money they did not expect to collect, even if it is not as much as they were owed. Then the repricer makes money by offering the patient, who does not understand that he or she could have received a much larger discount directly from the hospital. If the repricer also charges the patient a fee for the "savings" allegedly won, he or she has made money three times on the "savings."

Just as do the PPOs, the repricer has a financial interest in showing the recovering patient the highest charged rate possible. When you face a $60,000 hospital bill for your three-day stay, the repricer who says he or she can save you $20,000 sounds like a hero. Never mind that the insurance plan owned by your neighbor only pays the PPO $28,000 for those services. You will never know, if you must pay the bill yourself – the repricer did you a disservice.

Shhhhh! It's a secret

PPOs are shrouded in secrecy. Insurance companies execute proprietary secret contracts with their PPO network of physicians and hospitals. The contracts stipulate that the medical provider cannot share the details with anyone.

Individuals and employers that pay for a PPO health insurance plan only know the premium amount they pay: They know nothing about how much the carrier pays to the medical provider. In those cases when the carrier does show claims experience to the client, it usually does not include the actual net price paid to the providers.

Making this more complicated, an insurance carrier often has more than one network – and may have dozens. Each PPO network receives a different "discount." Therefore, the same insurance company can pay the same physician a different amount based on the identical service in the network in which the patient is enrolled.

Let's say Dr. Marvel is part of a PPO network called "Few Doctors," and another offered by the same insurance company called "Many Doctors." The insurance company pays Marvel $527.53 in the Many Doctor Network – but $705.92 in the Few Doctors Network. The person paying the insurance pays more premium for the Few Doctors Network and less premium for the Many Doctors Network – but gets

Rigged: How Insurance Ruined Health Care

the same level and quality of service. The amount paid to the same medical provider can vary by 1,000 percent, depending on which network is used by the patient. Usually the price variance has nothing to do with the quality of care.

What is the true price? It's close to impossible to know the true price, because there is no price transparency from the patient's point of view, and the insurance companies swear the providers to secrecy.

Health insurance companies want us to believe that these discounts benefit us and that we could not get those rates without their PPO networks. This is, however, a stark form of price-fixing where a third party decides what to pay for the patient, and the patient is not involved in approving the price. Any student of economics knows that price fixing increases the price of something, and eventually lead to shortages. Pre-negotiated PPO "discounts" are no different than other more open forms of price fixing.

Even in the end

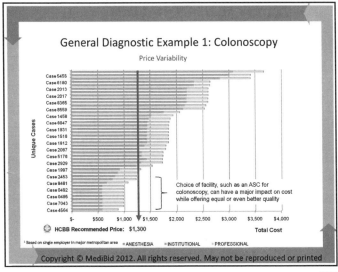

Rigged: How Insurance Ruined Health Care

The diagram above shows that providers have accepted prices ranging from $900 to $3,600 from the same insurance company's various PPO network for the same colonoscopy in the city of Nashville. But the patient has no idea his or her insurance company pays $900 or $3,600. (Actually most of these dollars pay only the facility fees, and the physicians' services are often paid separately.)

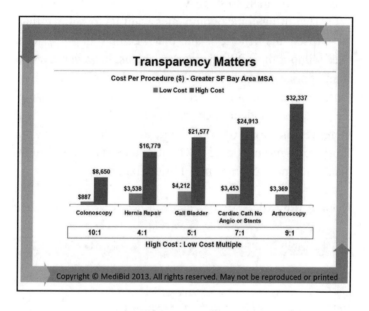

The above diagram shows an even greater variance in pricing for multiple procedures in the San Francisco Bay area.

As you can see, a patient with a PPO insurance policy has very little control over the price of his or her health care policy. Even with a high deductible plan, where the patient pays the first dollar cost, there is no patient price control in a PPO. MediCrats like all this secrecy about prices – it puts them more in charge, and it increases costs.

Rigged: How Insurance Ruined Health Care

Insurance companies do not tell you about the huge differences in what they pay for your medical care. They emphasize instead the 40-55 percent discounts they say they are winning for you. If they told you about the 400 to 1,000 percent difference in what they pay the same providers in different networks they know you would have a fit.

This formula drives up prices

When the chargemaster price is greater, the network "discounts" are inflated. The actual amount paid to the physicians or hospitals, on average, might be a fair or inflated price. The patient, however, cannot tell whether the discount really reduces prices.

Instead, the PPOs are huge profit centers in their own right. Most usually charge an access fee that can vary from a few dollars per month per person, to $15 per person or even more each month. Given that nearly 200 million American residents own private health insurance, these access fees can generate billions of dollars each year for the insurance companies that feature PPOs.

Another way that many PPOs profit is by showing one price on your EOB, which is in turn debited towards the employer's claims account, but pays a lower net cost to the physician or hospital.

Let's review: The medical provider sends a bill to the PPO at the insurance company. The insurance company then re-prices the bill to show the negotiated rate – often near 50 percent of the billed price. You see this on your Explanation of Benefits as the allowable rate. You may pay a portion of the bill depending on your deductible or co-insurance.

If you receive your insurance from an employer, the employer may be self-insured (sometimes called self-funded). This means the employer pays the cost of claims not paid by the employee. Any money owed the medical provider after the discount and your co-insurance or deductible is paid by your employer. To protect themselves from huge claims, employers buy "stop-loss insurance" – it pays the balance of the claims about above the stop-loss amount. If an employer is self-funded through a major insurance company – as opposed to a Third-Party Administrator (TPA) – the company often pools all of the company's claims above a certain amount, rather than using stop loss insurance. Depending on the pooling level, this could increase your costs because you are responsible for more of the claims.

Your employer also might provide fully-insured coverage. Under these policies, instead of the employer paying directly, the insurance company pays the provider, and the employer pays an insurance premium each month.

Yet, there are more mysteries surrounding the payment. It is possible that the employer will pay the bill but the provider receives a lesser amount. This happens when the claim is "down-coded" – meaning the billing codes are changed to a less expensive procedure – or it could be denied after the fact. The bills may be changed during a future audit. Sometimes the employer receives an additional bill. During 2012, the Blue Cross company of Michigan lost a case regarding "undisclosed hidden fees."

In a self-insured plan, the administrator has a fiduciary duty to protect the plan owner's assets. In the case listed above, Calhoun County vs. BCBS of Michigan, the federal court found Blue Cross had been engaging in prohibited transactions under the federal statute known as ERISA – (The Employee Retirement Income Security Act) by adding hidden undisclosed fees which drive up costs, called "Self-Dealing."

Rigged: How Insurance Ruined Health Care

When Texas teachers organized a way to share the cost of hospital bills in 1929 they created Blue Cross. In 1939, physicians organized Blue Shield as a way for people to pre-pay major medical expenses. Since then the health insurance industry has become a financial juggernaut, not only paying nearly $1 trillion a year in health care claims, but very often controlling how physicians and hospitals deliver health care – the perfect example of the Golden Rule: He who has the gold makes the rules. Health insurance MediCrats have amassed great power.

One of the ways HMOs sold themselves was to provide preventive care at low cost so that people would remain healthier. As a result, after the HMO Act of 1973 had passed, health insurance companies seem to have adopted the idea that medical care is simply an inconvenient cousin of health care. Prior to 1966, the most common insurance owned by most people was medical and hospital care. We were responsible for caring for our personal health, and paying the attendant cost.

Today, we purchase a product called health care, but few people know what that means or understand its implications. Health care is basically a series of payments, co-pays, deductibles, and co-insurance which finances our medical care. As used today, health care refers to the means of financing medical care. States, and now the federal government, require insurance companies to offer a long list of benefits: this includes payment for contraception, wigs, alcohol counseling, maternity, and many more services. These "health plans" include many "benefits" that you might not have ever purchased in your lifetime, especially if you had the freedom to decline these purchases government forces on you. Governments use laws and regulations to force you to spend money you might not have chosen to spend.

Rigged: How Insurance Ruined Health Care

Since the cost of health care is based on the price of medical care services and products, it cannot be controlled as long as health care itself is the product. It requires providing financial tools to make the price of care both transparent and important to individuals and have them pay at least some of the cost of their own medical care.

There are new answers to the pricing problem

The solution should start with individual patients, not with massive insurance and provider systems. Individuals have much greater bargaining power than the large health care entities. The PPOs, HMOs, and other forms of "health plans" want you to believe you cannot do this alone, but they are wrong.

A provider network must accept everyone that the insurance company has enrolled in their PPO. An individual patient, however, has the power to say NO. Think about it. NO is one of the most powerful negotiating words in our English vocabulary.

What if you could find the information you need about a health care provider or a procedure before spending your money? What if you could tell a physician NO when you review his or her price schedule and the services offered? What if you could choose the hospital, surgical center, or clinic you preferred, instead of the one your PPO requires? What if you could say YES to your choice and NO to the PPO?

This negotiating power is already available through MediBid. You can solicit bids from the nation's top medical providers or overseas providers before committing to the one of your choice. This is a powerful tool.

Some insurance administrators (called Third-Party Administrations – TPAs) have designed new ways of paying for care that are patient-centered – a Medicare allowable plan. As Chapter 11 explains in more depth, with this type of plan a referenced price is established that can be made transparent to both the patient and the provider. Then the patient can make an informed decision basing his or her choice on all factors, including the price of services.

One of the great advantages of a Medicare plus percentage insurance plan is that you can go to any willing medical provider. You are not chained to a PPO network. More importantly, it allows you to negotiate a cash price, which PPO networks do not.

In another chapter you will see how state medical boards affect pricing in their own states. This makes a service in one state far more expensive than the same service in a neighboring state. In Minnesota, for instance, you will go to a specialty clinic for a colonoscopy, while in Wisconsin you can receive the same test in a doctor's office. The savings in Wisconsin can be dramatic.

How to anger a MediCrat and save money, too

The PPO networks also incentivizes individuals to spend more money and increase the price of health care. This is done, in part, by how the PPO uses co-insurance and co-pays. Compare a colonoscopy provided by an in-network PPO to an "out-of-network" provider in Minnesota or Wisconsin. This example is representative of actual differences:

The in-network price in Minnesota may be $2,500, while the price in Wisconsin is $1,200 – but it is out-of-network for the Minnesotan. Let's assume the health plan pays 80 percent of the cost for in-network services and 50 percent of out-of-network services.

In this example, the individual's portion in Minnesota (in-network) would be $500, but it would be $600 in Wisconsin (out-of-network). This reduces the incentive for a patient to drive to Wisconsin to save money.

Consider the individual who receives insurance from a self-insured employer. The in-network cost for the employer is far greater than the out-of-network price. In Minnesota, the employee pays $500, but the employer pays $2,000. If the employee had chosen to go to Wisconsin and pay the $600, the employer's share would only be $600.

The employee has no personal incentive to drive the extra miles to Wisconsin. It would cost $100 more out of pocket, plus more time and expensive gasoline.

What is needed is a way to reward the employee for saving money for the employer. At MediBid you find such a plan – called "Reverse co-pay." MediBid provides a financial incentive to employees to reduce the cost of care paid by the employer. In the example above, instead of the employer paying $2,000 for its share of the bill – and the employee paying $500 – the reverse co-pay pays the employee $100 for choosing a Wisconsin provider. The company pays the $1,200 procedure price, and $100 to the employee – a total cost of $1,300 instead of the $2,000 under a traditional PPO plan. MediBid shops thousands of procedures and allows employers to set up MediBid networks saving 35 percent or more on their health insurance premiums.

The Affordable Care Act of 2010 defined a colonoscopy as preventive care. The new, very expensive health plans required by the ACA mandated that insurance covers 100 percent of the fee for preventive care. Yet, there are at least 14,000 other procedures where the reverse co-pay could save employers and employees money, give the patient more control over providers, improve health care, and reduce total spending. As Congress continues to "reform" health care finance, even colonoscopies might become an optional service requiring co-pays.

A better deductible idea

PPOs can reduce premiums by increasing the deductibles on their health plans. This means patients pay more of their own bills out-of-pocket. These plans have become increasingly popular to control insurance costs, and to try to engage the patient in making better spending choices. This idea, unfortunately, can have the exact opposite effect.

Over time, the deductible amounts have increased at the same time that the premiums have increased. A high deductible plan with a $500 a month premium costs a great deal less than a low-deductible plan with an $900 premium. Yet, just a few years ago that $500 premium was $150. The individual now pays far more for prepaid medical care cost, and the employer pays a greater premium. This creates a "death spiral" in which younger, healthier individuals refuse to purchase insurance, while less healthy and older individuals are buying ever-more expensive coverage with higher deductibles."

Another common tactic is what insurance agents call "chasing the deductible." This happens when the agent and/or carrier raises the deductible level each year to hold down premium increases. Too often, healthier and younger employees start to drop their insurance as the deductibles increase, no longer seeing the value of their insurance. When these younger healthier employees drop coverage, it leaves more unhealthy employees on the insurance plan. This simply accelerates the premium increases as the claims experience of the plan gets out of control. This creates yet another spike in premiums to cover the sicker enrollees – it becomes almost impossible to break this cycle. This is called "adverse selection."

A new type of deductible is emerging. Instead of an annual deductible, this new plan would use a monthly deductible. This concept forces individuals to act like consumers each month. It also allows for lower-cost, more affordable coverage for younger, healthier individuals – and everyone else. Instead of having a huge annual deductible, which for lower income workers simply acts as a barrier to care, the smaller, yet more frequent monthly deductible encourages them to get medical care they need early, instead of delaying medical care while the condition worsens, causing ultimately greater medical bills.

Another emerging idea would allow employers to share 50 percent of the cost on first dollar health care expenses with their employees. This would reduce the cost of insurance and give the employee an incentive to spend money more carefully.

Additional alternatives

The market price of anything could be defined as the highest price people are willing to pay to acquire or use something, and the lowest price a provider or producer is willing to accept. In a free market, those that provide products and services set their own prices, but always with an eye on the competition. The individual that pays for the products or services makes the ultimate judgment on market prices – saying NO or YES with their hard-earned dollars. These elements, however, do not exist in our health care insurance system where others – called third parties – set the prices. The third party pays the bills and sets the price with the provider. The individual patient has almost no control over the price of care, and in a PPO, very little control over which physician or hospital to use. This system will never solve our health care financing crisis. It could be argued that if a hospital accepts what Medicare pays for a service, that is the real, true market price.

Nearly all government attempts to reform health care fail, and a primary reason is they try to fix what does not work by repeating what does not work. We need a new approach.

Chapter 1 includes a quote from a 1919 issue of The Insurance Monitor, and it is worth repeating here:

> ...the opportunities for fraud [in health insurance] upset all statistical calculations...Health and sickness are vague terms open to endless construction. Death is clearly defined, but to say what shall constitute such loss of health as will justify insurance compensation is no easy task.

It is proper for health insurance to pay medical providers a reasonable price for their services. PPOs, however, do not produce reasonable rates – they create a wide range of prices without transparency.

The new way of crafting insurance policies must allow for price transparency and for individuals to purchase health care services and products based on their personal preference. An insurance plan that pays providers a percentage above the Medicare rate would accomplish this goal. A Florida court set a precedent for this in a case involving a disputed hospital bill. The court eventually ruled that a fair price to settle that dispute was the Medicare rate plus 20 percent. Whether a local health care market would agree to Medicare plus 20 percent or to some greater factor above Medicare is already being proven by MediBid every day. We need a new way to pay for health care, and this would be a great alternative.

To make any patient-controlled health care payment system work, however, we need additional tools. MediBid.com is such a tool. It is here that the patient can predetermine the cost of care and make informed decisions about where to spend health care dollars.

Combining a monthly deductible insurance plan with one that pays providers a reasonable rate; a plan that encourages paying a reduced price; a plan that lets the patient cross state lines to get the best value; a plan that gives the patient the ability to see the price ahead of time; these are the elements that would create a market-based plan and will lead to a marketplace for medicine.

Politicians cannot create the right environment for health care; they can only dismantle the barriers to a true health care marketplace. The business of politics, however, is rewarding friends and campaign contributors, and creating an army of MediCrats who owe their livelihoods to the politicians is the natural outcome. It is this mix of politics and influence that created and perpetuates the health care crisis.

Solving the health care pricing crisis requires a strong dose of American entrepreneurial energy – and cutting away the cancer of socialism, fascism, and statism. The time of the PPO is passing, and individual control should replace it.

MediPlan: A new wrinkle

Ultimately, true insurance is good insurance, and is an effective method for sharing risk. Most typical pre-paid medical plans include services that are legitimately covered by true medical insurance. These include emergency room visits and hospital inpatient surgeries. MediBid created health insurance that covers just these necessary events and we label this the Catastrophic Minimum Essential Coverage (CAT-MEC) Plan.

No one can shop for the best value in emergency room care in advance, and you certainly can't do it in an ambulance on the way to the hospital. As a result, the CAT-MEC Plan pays the hospital at network prices. We urge employers to pay the premium for 100 percent of the cost of the CAT-MEC plan. This gives all insured employees access to base coverage.

A second tier of coverage is also offered under the MediPlan. It pays physicians, hospitals, and other medical providers a fee based on what Medicare would pay, plus 30 or 50 percent, depending on the region. These covered procedures tend to be less costly, and usually MediBid – or the individual – can negotiate a cash price. This part of the coverage also pays the cost of other medical needs such as generic prescriptions, outpatient procedures, lab work, imaging, doctors' office visits, etc. Employers should share the premium cost for this health plan with their employees.

A combination of these tiers, when combined with other concepts outlined in this chapter, can create health insurance that is compliant with the new federal health care law – ACA – yet remains affordable and cost effective.

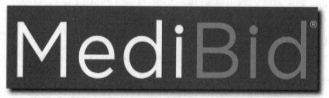

The marketplace for medicine.

The best way to finance health care is to know the price before you buy it. At MediBid.com you can find the greatest value simply by asking physicians and surgeons to bid on your care.

Chapter 8

Financing Health Care

Imagine yourself in a car showroom. You are staring at a gray sedan. This is not really the car you want, but when you came into the showroom, you had set a budget. You planned to spend no more than $19,000 on a new car. The gray car lists for $18,500.

You cannot keep your eyes off a red sports car sitting nearby. "This is what I really want," you think to yourself. Then you looked at the sticker price, and got sticker shock -- $29,000.

A salesman stood to the side watching you. At the right moment, he walked up and said, "She is a beauty, isn't she?"

After carefully quizzing you, the salesman had everything he needed to close a sale. "Let me show you the numbers," he said as you sat down together. Within minutes, the salesman showed you could buy the red sports car for "less money" than the gray sedan: in fact, for $125 per month less. He had stretched the payments out over six years, instead of the four years you originally requested.

Many, really most people, buy cars in this manner. Real estate agents understand this, too.

Rigged: How Insurance Ruined Health Care
"You Can Afford It"

The crash of home prices in 2007 and for several years following may have changed this scenario a bit, but it is characteristic of how Americans have bought homes during the last 20 years. Of course, you would never do it this way: but your neighbor probably did.

You need a 1,200 square foot home. It would meet your needs. Where you live, a house like this with a double garage, sells for $210,000. You have saved $10,000 for a down payment. "No problem," says the real estate agent. "I can show you many homes in that price range." Then the agent pauses and asks, "If you could get the home you really want, what would it look like?" The home you describe is two stories, with a three-car garage, on an acre of land.

After looking at three 1,200 square foot homes, you started to become discouraged. They were okay, but not when you really want. The realtor turned the corner and stopped in front of your dream house. "Let's walk through it," she said. In less than five minutes you felt you really wanted it.

"Now, this is more than you expected to pay, of course. This house sells for $319,000, and that's a bargain. The previous owner died, and the family wants to sell the house quickly." She looked you in the eye and added, "I am certain we can make the numbers work."

Within 10 minutes, she showed you that you would need about $5,000 more for closing costs. These costs, however, could be rolled into the mortgage. Here is the "great part:" By stretching out the mortgage over 30 years, instead of the 15-year plan you wanted, your principal and interest payments were quite affordable. Even with the taxes and insurance added, your combined income made it possible to qualify.

Congratulations! You now have a place to park the new red sports car in your new three car garage. For as long as you have a job, you should be able to keep them both.

We buy health care the same way

Prepaid health insurance hides the true cost of services and products. In this, health insurance agents are somewhat like the car salesmen and real estate agent.

This author has been in the insurance business for more than 20 years, and I have still never heard an insurance client who owns a prepaid health plan ask, "How much would it cost for me to have…" and then name a procedure. "How much is a physical?" "What does a blood test cost?"

"So, if I get a new knee, what is the total cost of the pre-op physical and blood work, anesthesiologist, surgical team, hospital, physical therapy, and everything else I have to pay?" No one has asked me these questions.

"How much is my monthly insurance premium?" This is the question my clients ask me. It is the same question you asked the car salesman when you bought the red sports car. "What's my monthly payment?" The actual price is masked by focusing on the monthly payment. (Not surprisingly, a certain number of Americans refuse to buy health insurance because it costs more than their car payment. Never mind the fact that a minor illness can turn into a $10,000-$15,000 expense overnight.)

Think of health insurance in the same way you think of a car payment or house payment. There is one major difference, however: car payments and house payments are held steady over the term of the contract. Health insurance premiums tend to go up every year, but for most people, so does their medical risk. Even at this, their primary concern is the monthly premium, not the actual cost of health care.

Rigged: How Insurance Ruined Health Care

Health "insurance" is simply a way to finance medical care. The actual cost of care really does not matter to most people.

In the last two decades, monthly health insurance premiums have become the single most expensive budget item for many families. From $200 a month to insure a family several years ago, it is not uncommon to find family premiums in excess of $2,200 a month today.

Monthly premiums have become increasingly less affordable. As a result, the politicians decided to step in once again and ignore the real problem: the price of health care services. Instead, the politicians focused on reforming the financing of health care through an attempt to control monthly health insurance premiums.

Insurance premiums finance health care spending. Spending is the total cost of medical care times utilization. The more an individual uses health care services, the more they spend. The more they spend, the greater their monthly premium grows.

When we buy house insurance, car insurance, or life insurance, we don't run home and dream of ways to "use" the insurance. We pay our relatively small premiums for years and hope we never have to make a claim. Health "insurance" is different. We pay a hefty premium every month and try to find ways to "use" it. In fact, we feel cheated if we don't.

How the politicians responded

The Affordable Care Act of 2010 (ACA) gave the federal Secretary of Health and Human Services (DHHS) power to limit insurance premiums. The ACA did this at least two ways: 1) It gave explicit power to the secretary, working with states, to set limits on premium increases. 2) It created and provided enforcement for the Medical Loss Ratio (MLR). We wrote in detail about the MLR in an earlier chapter.

The ACA allowed the federal Secretary of Health and Human services to review health insurance premium rates. The law gave the federal government access to as much as $50 million to grant to each state to help the state monitor and control health insurance rate increases. This new federal MediCratic oversight reduced the power of states to regulate health insurance within their borders, and moved decision-making to Washington, D.C. In states that already had aggressive insurance review processes in place, the new law added yet another level of MediCrats.

Each time a MediCrat has to review medical processes or insurance policies, the cost for you ticks upward. Someone has to pay for the additional review. It will be you, through higher insurance premium, or someone else, through greater taxes.

If today you were thinking about having a physical, but you knew you would have to write a check for $750, it is possible you would wait. You might, instead, spend some time thinking about your body and how it feels. If you sense there has been no change since the last physical, you might choose to wait another year. If you see you have gained weight, you might go on a diet. If you feel weak and sluggish, you might begin exercising. These lifestyle changes can be done at no expense.

Here is an example of how the Medical Loss Ratio might increase your cost. In most states, and under the ACA, your insurance policy will pay 100 percent of the cost of a physical – you don't even have to pay a co-pay. Under these conditions, you would have the physical. The insurance company would need to add $187.50 on top of the $750 so it can get its 20 percent for administrative cost. The physical you do not need will cost you (or your employer or taxpayers) $937.50. How should you feel about this?

If you pay $1,000 a month for prepaid health care (health insurance) chances are you will get the physical. You feel entitled to it. Your monthly premium is the way you finance the physical you may or may not need.

To further cut cost

Since the ACA, and 45 years of health insurance evolution, refuses to address the negative incentives of prepaid health care, CMS and insurance companies use MediCrats to force down the cost of care by dictating how much physicians and hospitals will be paid. Renewed Congressional efforts to replace and reform the ACA continue to resolve this issue. Among the problems this creates, perhaps the most serious is a critical, pending shortage of physicians.

> According to updated statistics from the Association of American Medical Colleges, the United States faces a "projected shortfall of between 40,800 and 104,900 physicians by 2030." The wide swing in the projected shortfall is because of the variety of conditions that could occur over time – yet even at 40,800 (the low end), the shortfall is concerning. The extremes in the range are unlikely, but a mid-range estimate of 73,000 too few physicians is at least a moderate crisis.[1]

As the number of available physicians and surgeons continues to fall, those that remain will most likely go one of two ways: Some will practice under contract with a mas-

---

[1] Dall, Tim, Ritashree Chakrabarti, Will Iacobucci, Alpana Hansari, and Terry West. "The Complexities of Physician Supply and Demand: Projections from 2015 to 2030 - 2017 Update." Association of American Medical Colleges, February 28, 2017. https://aamc-black.global.ssl.fastly.net/production/media/filer_public/a5/c3/a5c3d565-14ec-48fb-974b-99fafaeecb00/aamc_projections_update_2017.pdf.

sive, federally-controlled, Accountable Care Organization (ACO). As ACO doctors, these physicians may settle for less income but also work under more top-down control. Other physicians and surgeons will opt for new free market practice options, and will be the preferred choice of those who 1) are willing to pay and 2) cannot get the quality of care they seek from an ACO.

This presents an opportunity for both non-ACO physicians and patients. For the physician, it increases the opportunity to be an entrepreneur and to define the services and quality he or she will deliver. Non-ACO physicians will be freed from the constraints imposed on them by insurance and government MediCrats. Patients that choose non-ACO physicians will retain the opportunity to visit a professional willing to spend quality time with them, so that together, the patient and physician can decide the best course of action. The physician will empower and educate the patient, rather than simply medicate them. Remember, an ACO doctor is accountable to the payer, while a private doctor works for the patient.

No matter whether physicians choose to work in ACOs or private practice, patients will pay more for their services. This is always the end result of a shortage of supply.

Another way of dealing with the supply shortage, or to reduce the price of care, is to travel to locations where health care services can be delivered at less cost. This is often called "medical tourism."

You can travel if you have a mind to, and want to save money

Even with all the restrictions, it is possible to travel across state lines to save money on necessary health care procedures. Many people, in fact, are traveling to foreign countries for medical therapy and surgery. This is called "medical tourism."

Usually, medical tourism is linked to travel to a foreign country. When traveling to a foreign country, the individual not only receives surgical and medical services, but takes time to enjoy the host country. The savings can be significant – even enormous.

Overseas hospitals bring other strengths to the table, and not only in their pricing and transparency. They tend not to practice defensive medicine – prescribing tests and processes to protect the physician against a potential lawsuit. Foreign medical providers can sometimes perform procedures not available in the U.S. due to the long-time delays imposed by the FDA, and tens or hundreds of millions of dollars required to receive FDA approval

Medical tourism, however, can be accessed without traveling abroad.

At MediBid.com, a patient that needs a medical procedure may find a physician in their own state willing to do it for less than the hometown doctor. Sometimes it's a matter of simply crossing state lines to receive medical care. Some medical procedures may require hospitalization in one state, while they can be performed in a doctors' office in a neighboring state. This can produce significant savings. MediBid.com has found a way to pair doctors with patients based on price, quality, and specific procedures. Patients can indicate the procedure they need, and a host of doctors will bid on providing that service.

Each state has its own unique characteristics that affect the price of health care. For instance, it costs more to build a hospital in California than Arizona, due to earthquake retrofitting, and environmental regulations. This adds hundreds of dollars to a hospitalization in California that can be saved by traveling to nearby Arizona.

An orthopedic surgeon in one state may charge $25,000 complete for a new knee. In another state, the price might be $12,000 – or less. A hospital in India may charge $7,500 for the same procedure.

Medical malpractice insurance has made health care more unaffordable across the country. Some U.S. states have clamped down on frivolous medical liability lawsuits to reduce the cost of medical care and attract more doctors. California, Texas, and Tennessee for instance, have placed limits on damages a person can collect from a medical malpractice lawsuit. This has resulted in making the price of medical procedures somewhat less expensive in these states than they would be otherwise. It also means that an individual could travel to Texas to save money on a medical or surgical procedure or diagnostic test. An increasingly large number of people are doing so.

Using the services of MediBid.com, a patient in Kansas City might find an MRI priced as little as $350 or as much as $1,850. If the quality and service is the same, and the patient has a Health Savings Account (HSA), the patient may prefer to save $1,500 on the same MRI.

DeLoitte and Touche, the National Consulting firm, suggests that medical tourism will grow 35 percent per year in the years ahead. Two reasons for this growth are 1) the lack of pricing transparency from traditional United States medical providers, and, 2) no real competition among medical providers. Medical tourism, then, becomes a motivation for American medical providers to make their prices and procedures more transparent. We must, however, guard against the MediCrats getting involved in this competitive pricing system and ruining medical tourism.

Rigged: How Insurance Ruined Health Care

While it makes sense economically to grow wheat in Saskatchewan, make stereos in Japan, and make clothing in China, medical care is what we do best in the United States. There is a prominent place in the market for medical tourism. We should, however, guard against completely outsourcing the health care of U.S. patients, and the best way is to redesign United States' health care to maximize our dollars.

Allow doctors to set their own rates and compete

Years ago, doctors knew the price they charged for medical procedures, and after a patient consultation, could agree with the patient on the best course of care.

Today, clinics and hospitals bill medical procedures at grossly inflated prices. Medical providers make care seem so out of reach that consumers perceive health care as unaffordable. Consumers then purchase a health plan based on an "affordable" monthly premium, or travel overseas for care.

The love/hate relationship between hospitals and third-party payers is very interesting. Remember, it was hospitals that invented Blue Cross, and even as Blue Cross spun off and grew on its own, they are still addicted to the money.

Once everyone has a health plan, they use it to purchase covered medical procedures, and if the procedure is not covered, they threaten to sue the insurance company anyway. Reformers try to decrease the cost of health care financing by capping customer service budgets and reducing transparency, leaving all medical decisions in the hands of MediCrats. They also encourage increased consumption by preferring lower deductibles so that more people will purchase these procedures. Then they fix the price of medical care and cap physicians' earnings so that doctors have to churn out more medicine.

Both drug and health insurance companies benefit from this perverse system of health care financing while the public loses. The public has been shielded from the high cost of medical care because of their health plans. When those plans cost a family $499 a month, they may have complained, but loved the access it gave them to care – whether or not they needed it. Since January 1, 2014, as the ACA health insurance reforms kicked in. those monthly premiums soared, in some states by more than 300 percent in three years. Today, individuals and families that do not qualify for a taxpayer-subsidized health plan, are getting sticker shock. Even so, because of the zero down, monthly financing scheme – called health insurance premiums – they continue to spend on care without knowing the price. Medical tourism, whether overseas or domestic, is a response to all these perverse market incentives.

The only way to achieve sustainable medical costs is to allow physicians to set their own prices (based on what patients will pay) and allow them to compete across state lines and international borders based on price and quality. MediBid.com offers those opportunities without changing any state or federal laws. Americans must reject health care finance as it has been pitched and recognize that insurance is for unexpected losses.

Chapter 9

Health Insurance as Insurance

Hall of Fame football coach, Vince Lombardi, while holding a football in his hand, started each year's practices with this simple phrase: "Gentlemen, this is a football."

Before anyone can play football, they must know what it is. They must also acknowledge that the game they are playing is American football, not "Sports." Congress and the MediCrats claim they are giving us "health care reform," but in reality, almost all their focus is on health care payment systems. Before we can reform health "care" we should understand health insurance.

Health Insurance 101

At its simplest, insurance is a way for people to share the financial risk of an unpredictable loss. "Insurance" is not people saving together to pay for expenses they expect or hope to incur. As discussed in the previous chapter, insurance isn't a product which we hope to use. When we buy car insurance, home insurance, or life insurance we don't hope to "use" it, but health insurance has been designed contrary to insurance principles. Perhaps, this is why it does not work very well.

Rigged: How Insurance Ruined Health Care

When you buy a car, you can buy auto insurance and you might choose to buy a prepaid maintenance plan – they are two different things. Auto insurance does not pay for routine maintenance, and prepaid maintenance plans do not pay for auto body repairs. You purchase auto insurance just in case someone crashes into you, or you crash into someone or something. Auto insurance pays to repair the car's body and mechanical systems if damaged in an accident. You purchase a prepaid maintenance plan to cover the cost of expected wear and tear – these plans are quite expensive.

If auto insurance also paid for routine maintenance, it would be extremely expensive. Chances are the cost would exceed the value of the automobile.

Insurance purchased to protect human beings from unexpected financial loss could be labeled "health" insurance. More appropriately, this type of insurance should be called major medical or hospital insurance, as it was before the mid-1960s. Hospital and major medical insurance always carried relatively high deductibles. People of that day did not expect to use their insurance, in fact if they did it meant they had suffered a serious illness or injury --no one wanted that to happen.

Prior to the mid-1960s, people paid for routine medical expense – "maintenance" – out of their pocket, or savings in much the same way we pay for gas and oil changes for our car today. They paid the physician in cash or wrote them a check (or maybe a dozen eggs). Everyone understood how this worked. Everyone expected everyone else, and themselves, to pay their own way. If an individual needed help, families or the community found ways to provide medical care.

With prepaid medical "insurance," however, people have come to expect routine medical care to be paid by their health plan. In fact, the term "health plan" actually describes prepaid health care. It really does attempt to act like an auto maintenance plan. Why should we be surprised that it is becoming more unaffordable?

There is one other similarity between auto and health insurance that we should discuss, and one significant difference. Under a routine maintenance plan, the contract (insurance policy) explains what is covered and what is not covered. At the auto repair shop, a service manager tells you which services the shop will do at no additional cost, and those for which you must pay more. The service manager and you are both subject to the contract.

With today's health plans, your physician and you are subject to the contract. The health plan contract tells the physician what services are covered, and sets the price of services. The physician must convince a health plan company MediCrat to deviate or extend coverage for questionable services, rather than come to agreement with you. If you want services or products not covered by your health plan, there is nothing in your health plan to stop you from spending your own money. That is between you and your physician. An auto maintenance plan and health insurance, then, are similar in that only covered services are provided without extra expense, and are subject to a third party deciding which services you will receive and which you will not receive.

One extremely significant difference exists between auto and health insurance. Auto insurance will pay up to the cash value of a car if the damages exceed the car's value – it will never pay more than the car's value. It will not pay for repairs just because you want to keep the car, and prefer that it is fixed.

Human beings, most of us believe, should not be subject to a maximum dollar amount for health care services. We consider human life to be beyond a monetary value. Most of us reject the idea that a MediCrat or insurance contract should be able to set a maximum spending limit on our own health care. The ACA, however, planned to do this exact thing through the Independent Payment Advisory Board (IPAB): it is called rationing. The 15 members of the IPAB, appointed by the president, was designed so the Board would decide which services are covered and at what price. If the IPAB survives the latest round of health care reforms and is activated, and you are enrolled in a government health plan, you will not be making that determination – the IPAB will do it for you.

There is a better way

The good news is that until the day when we can throw off MediCratic medicine and health plans, there is something we can do. We do have the right to choose major medical and hospital insurance – called consumer directed health plans. These are like what were common prior to 1965, but with some exciting features.

You will see this demonstrated in Table 2 on the next page: "Adaptive Health care." It describes options that are available to you today. These options make far more sense than spending thousands of dollars a year for a health plan that provides services you neither need nor want.

First, you find an affordable health insurance policy. It features a high deductible of as much as $5,000 for an individual and $10,000 for a family. The insurance premium for this type of policy could be as much as 35 to 75 percent less than for a traditional health plan. The table below compares monthly premiums for traditional plans with high deductible plans, based on age.

Notice in Table 2 that the plan with a $5,000 single deductible costs 38 percent less than the plan with the $250

Table 2

	20/250/100% AMD2 w/NS (SM)	HSA5000/100% AEOS w/DT (SM)
	Platinum	Silver
	N/A	$450-$750
	TX_MC17	TX_MC18
	TXD17	TXD 18
	2	20
	01/00/CG	01/00/CG
	$737.54	$459.11
	$1,475.05	$918.22
	$1,475.08	$918
	$2,212.62	$1,377.33
	$8,850.48	$5,509.32
	$9,588.02	$5,968.43
	$18,438.50	$11,477.75
	100%	100%
	$8,850.48	$5,509.32
	$221,262.00	$137,733.00
	0.00%	0.00%
	1	1
	$0.00	$0.00
	12	12
	13	13
	12	12
	19	19
	31	31
	CHOICE	CHOICE
	Premier	H.S.A.
	$250 / NA	$5000 / NA
	$750 / NA	$10000 / NA

Rigged: How Insurance Ruined Health Care

Table 3

PLAN	A	B	C	D	E
Deductible	$ -	$ 250.00	$ 1,000.00	$ 3,000.00	$ 6,550.00
Family Deductible	$ -	$ 500.00	$ 2,000.00	$ 6,000.00	$ 13,100.00
Co Insurance	50%	80%	70%	50%	100%
Total Out Of Pocket	$ 7,150.00	$ 1,250.00	$ 4,000.00	$ 6,000.00	$ 6,550.00
Total Family OOP	$ 14,300.00	$ 2,500.00	$ 8,000.00	$ 12,000.00	$ 13,100.00
Co Pay	$ 60.00	$ 25.00	$ 25.00	$ 40.00	100% After Ded
Drug co pay	$20/50%	0/10/35/75/150	10/30/50/25%	20/40/60/20%	100% After Ded
Monthly Premium	$ 1,118.21	$ 1,378.53	$ 1,172.16	$ 1,016.76	$ 515.07
Total - OOP	$ 14,300.00	$ 2,500.00	$ 8,000.00	$ 12,000.00	$ 13,100.00
Annual Premium	$ 13,418.46	$ 16,542.36	$ 14,065.92	$ 12,201.12	$ 6,180.84
Maximum in a bad year	$ 27,718.46	$ 19,042.36	$ 22,065.92	$ 24,201.12	$ 19,280.84

Table 4

Contribution Limits

2018 Limits	Single	Family
Minimum Deductible	$1,350	$2,700
Maximum Out-of-Pocket	$6,650	$13,300
Contribution Limit	$3,450	$6,900
Catch-up Contribution (55 or older)	$1,000	$1,000

deductible. Table 3 on the previous page, compares the cost of premium for single coverage.

Ask yourself this question: "Why would I want to pay as much as $10,362 more per year than I had to pay?" You may worry that if you need health care services, and you have a high deductible, you will not have the money to purchase them. However, this makes no sense. The difference is, of course, that you must set aside the money you save on premium to pay up to the full deductible or any other out of pocket expense. Another way to look at it is that if you could own a plan with a $10,000 deductible for free, or a plan with a zero deductible for $10,362, which would you take?

The good news about out-of-pocket expenses is that the federal government gives you a way to do this using pre-tax dollars. Tax law allows you to deposit money into a Health Savings Account (HSA) subject to annual limits and other rules. Table 4 above shows that for 2018, an individual can deposit up to $3,450 into an HSA and pay no federal tax on it as long as it's used for approved expenses. A family can deposit up to $6,900 into its HSA per year. These deposit limits are related to the amount of deductible in your health insurance, and other factors. Additionally, 47 states also allow a state tax deduction on deposits. Call a qualified professional health insurance agent for details.

Employers have additional options to assist employees and maximize the advantage of their high deductible insurance and HSA. Employers can use a Health Reimbursement Arrangement (HRA) combined with the HSA in such a way as to reduce out of pocket expenses. This separates the high deductible health "insurance" from the routine health care expenses "extended warranty" so that utilization of routine care does not affect the cost of the insurance.

The result of owning an HSA combined with a high deductible health plan and an HRA is that you become more of a health care consumer. Since some of the money you spend on routine health care will come from your own HSA, you become more concerned about the price of medical services. You learn to shop for the best value on prescription medicine, durable medical equipment, medical supplies, and even physicians, surgeons, and hospitals.

> This is a true story: Dave, a 60-year old man, suffered from sleep apnea. The doctor prescribed a CPAP machine. Dave went to a medical supply company and found the model he wished to use. As the clerk wrote the order, Dave asked, "How much does this cost?" The question shocked the clerk, and she had no answer.
>
> Dave called the medical supply company's business office and asked the same question: "I have an HSA and high deductible insurance. Please, how much does this CPAP cost?"

"$200 a month on a 10-month lease," the business office manager said.

"But, I don't want to lease it. I want to buy it. How much does it cost?" Dave asked. This is how medical consumerism works. When you use your own money, you care about the price of durable medical devices.

"$1,395," the office manager said.

Dave bought the CPAP outright. In so doing, just in the first 10 months he saved $605. He never asked how much the company meant to charge him after 10 months, but he really did not care: he owned his own machine. Imagine the savings across the entire United States' health care system if this type of story could be repeated millions of times a day.

It is possible, however, that Dave could have done even better, and saved more if he had purchased it through the medical equipment portal at MediBid.com.

You have to buy smart

Earlier, you read about MediBid.com, the Marketplace for Medicine.

At MediBid.com, you can enter information about your medical condition and need, and the information is evaluated by thousands of prospective medical doctors. Among those that evaluate your need, someone will choose to bid on providing the service to you. When they do, they also provide you with a price for the service. You can review the training and experience of the medical professional in order to determine the quality of care he/she provides.

Once you have reviewed the various bids, you are free to contact the bidding physician or surgeon of your choice.

Rigged: How Insurance Ruined Health Care

You decide where to receive your medical services, and to the extent that you agree with the price quoted by the physician or surgeon, you also control the price you are willing to pay.

Dave, that 60-year old man that bought a CPAP machine, might very well have found a better price at MediBid.com, where medical suppliers are willing to provide bids for durable medical equipment. If Dave needed an MRI, CT scan, or other diagnostic test, he could stand to save hundreds of dollars, maybe even thousands, by posting his need at MediBid.com.

MediBid.com has physician and surgeon members from across the world, but the greatest number practice in the United States. This means that it is very possible for you to find the high-quality health care services you need, at a more affordable price, and not have to travel to distant land to receive them.

The overseas providers are often able to bring unique techniques, medical devices, and cutting-edge care processes into the operating room. Sometimes, this is because a procedure is not covered by insurance in the U.S. or not yet approved by a government agency. Yet, it is successfully performed overseas. Procedures such as High Intensity Focused Ultrasound (HIFU) for prostate cancer, or Hyperthermia for breast cancer, or even Heavy Proton Radiation for other types of cancer could be available overseas, but not in the U.S.

Some procedures are just more affordable abroad, and many overseas facilities look like Seven Star Resorts. They know how to cater to Americans. When you go for care abroad, they often have accommodations for your "significant other" as well, so you can make a wonderful vacation out of it.

Adaptive Healthcare: Less money, better care

Most of the unnecessary waste in health care comes from having third-party payers – health insurance companies and HMOs – decide what kind of health care we need, and then pay the insurance company MediCrats to pay physicians to provide it. In third grade math we learned that if you put four apples into a basket, you cannot take five out unless you steal someone else's apple. Low cost medical procedures performed with high frequency all cost money to administer. The cost for a MediCrat to write a check for a $65 office visit is no different than paying for a $25,000 surgery. The office visits are predictable, the surgeries are not.

Adaptive Healthcare starts with you owning a first dollar Health Savings Account (HSA). The employer and employee together deposit $125 per month into the HSA for those with single coverage. By the end of the year, they have deposited $1,500 (just above the 2018 minimum deductible needed according to IRS rules).

As you spend these funds on health care needs, you decide how and when to spend these dollars. Since it is your money, you are careful in how you spend it. Should your medical needs exceed $1,500 in a given calendar year, you dip into your Health Reimbursement Arrangement (HRA). The HRA acts much like a credit line established by the employer, but not used until the employee has already spent $1,500. The next $5,000 of medical expenses are covered by the employer out of the HRA.

The insurance company has found that only 20 percent of people spend their entire HSA in a year. Just 49 percent of employees exhaust their entire HRA. Using those assumptions, only two of 10 employees will even tap into the employer's HRA funds, and only one of those two will use all $5,000. If an employee should spend their $1,500 HSA and

Rigged: How Insurance Ruined Health Care

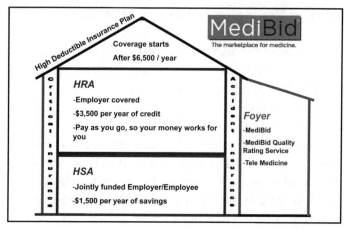

the $5,000 HRA, their high deductible health plan kicks in after $6,500 and covers 100 percent of medical expenses.

To protect those $6,500 of medical expenses, the insurance agent installs two different policies to reinsure the deductible: 1) Accident insurance to cover unexpected accidents or injuries up to $10,000, and 2) Critical Illness insurance to cover as many as 21 critical illnesses – heart attack, cancer, stroke, kidney failure etc. with a $10,000 tax free cash payout.

As we have addressed throughout this book, health care provider systems sadly lack price transparency, and competition among medical providers is quite limited. Safeway Foods studied price transparency, and estimated that knowing the price of care could save a company 16 percent of their health care costs. So on the front end of this plan we install a tool to help employees become educated, informed shoppers, and provide them access to MediBid.com. This allows employees to define their own criteria in shopping for health care services, and helps them to find a better price for that care.

All of these pieces combine to produce better health

Compare For Yourself

Old Managed Care
- $250/$500 Deductible
- 80% Coinsurance
- $25 Copay
- 0/10/35/75/150 Drugs
- $1,379 Premium

Adaptive Healthcare ©
- $125 HSA
- $104 HRA
- $39 CI
- $15 Foyer
- $515 Premium
- $798 Total
- $83,664 Annual Savings

Based on a group of 12 Employees in Texas
with an 8/1/2017 Start Date

care coverage at 42 percent lower cost. For example, a small company in Texas with 12 full time employees based on a August 1, 2017 start date has been able to reduce their premium cost from $16,548 per month to $9,576, an annual savings of $83,664. Imagine the health care savings all of us could enjoy if everyone did that!

The bottom line

No one wants to waste money on health care for insurance they don't need or want, and no one wants to pay more than they must. When someone else pays your medical bills, as is common to comprehensive, low deductible health plans, you do not worry about the cost of each service: you worry about the monthly premium, and it is becoming less affordable each day. When you pay some of your own medical bills, and purchase health "insurance" instead of prepaid health care, you save thousands on premium payments and thousands more when you need medical care.

The bottom line is that the best health care system is

the one controlled by you, as you work closely with the physician or surgeon of your choice. Your most fundamental property right is the right to your own body, and you need to be the one to decide what kind of care you want, not the MediCrats who want to regulate your health.

Health care does not need to be expensive, and does not need to be subject to high inflation. It is only because people have insisted that health "insurance" covers everything that it has become this way. If I asked you to imagine how much car insurance would cost if it covered gas and oil changes, you could imagine that. You would also know that if it did, we would all drive hummers and take very long drives every weekend.

Maybe insurance is the problem

"America hasn't had a free market in health insurance for decades. ...In a free market, prices are the Great Regulator."[1]

The United States' choice for paying the cost of health care breaks primarily along two lines. First, there are numerous health plans paid directly by governments – federal and state. And, there are premium-paid, commercial insurance politics - health insurance. Both have this in common: They hide the price of care from patients so that individuals have little to no incentive to fight for a lower price of their care. Individuals have no skin in the game.

The U.S. system of health "insurance" as we know it, is the primary enabler for waste of money in the health care system. Americans expect to access any and all care they believe they need, when they want it, at someone else's ex-

---

[1] Hall, Jon. "Articles: The 'Free Market' and Universal Health Care," April 9, 2017. http://www.americanthinker.com/articles/2017/04/the_free_market_and_universal_healthcare.html.

pense. Politicians know there is a limit to what people will pay, in taxes and for premiums, and have begun to clamp down on care using increasingly MediCrat-heavy tactics. In this way, insurance is ruining health care.

Rigged: How Insurance Ruined Health Care

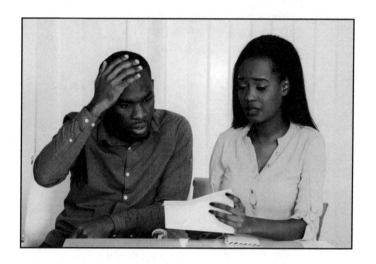

CHAPTER 10

HOW INSURANCE RUINED HEALTH CARE

Politics, def.

poli Latin, for many. *tics* are bloodsuckers.

Merriam-Webster's more traditional definition:
  a : the art or science of government
  b : the art or science concerned with guiding or influencing governmental policy
  c : the art or science concerned with winning and holding control over a government

For the purposes of this chapter, our definition and Merriam-Webster's fit perfectly together.

Economists call United States' health care finance a "complex economic system." A complex economic system "…sees the economy not as a system in equilibrium, but as one in motion, perpetually constructing itself anew."[1] Such a system is hard to control since grass roots' folks prefer liv-

---

[1] "Complexity Economics." Wikipedia, April 8, 2017.
https://en.wikipedia.org/w/index.php?title=Complexity_economics&oldid=774412569.

ing their own lives as they see fit, taking risks as they chose to do so, and living with the unpredictable nature of human behavior. The fact that everyone is an individual making individual decisions does not, however, discourage MediCrats from trying to control individual health care.

Since the mid-1960s, the United States health care system has leaned on MediCrats at CMS, Health Maintenance Organizations (HMO), Preferred Provider Organizations (PPO), and Managed Care Organizations (MCO) to control spending on health care. The health plans that MediCrats and politicians have designed to support these systems distort the financing of health care by placing a veil of complexities between the payer and the patient. Instead of considering the price of care as a contributing factor in decisions about purchasing care, MediCrats have attempted to make price irrelevant to patients.

The false concept under which payment plans operate is that enough science, data, and wisdom exist at the highest management levels to enforce the best decisions on individuals, who simply want to reduce their pain and suffering, and see their lives extended.

The reality is that how health "insurance" leaves the patient out of the health care finance decision is ruining health care.

Health Care Crisis, or Maybe Not

In 1959, *The New York Times* lamented that 22 percent of Americans lacked any kind of health insurance. Of course, insurance at that time meant major medical and hospital insurance, far different from today. Despite the media lament, there were not widespread reports of people dying on the streets for lack of medical care – county hospitals and charity care were available for those unable to pay their way.

Rigged: How Insurance Ruined Health Care

The cost of care in the 1950s was affordable for almost everyone. Patients paid doctors and hospitals directly for nearly all medical care, and in some places, they paid with food, firewood, or favors instead of money. The insurance they may have owned took care of catastrophic expenses. Insurance had not yet ruined the pricing system.

The 1960s' budding health care "crisis," however, served an important political purpose. It fueled Congress' bipartisan passage of Medicare and Medicaid in 1965. In the run-up to this revolution in health care pricing, pundits solemnly reported about widows being forced to eat dog food because the cost of their medical care left them destitute, or they had to forgo the care they needed.

After Congress passed Medicare and Medicaid, the U.S. has continued to experience one health care "crisis" after another, until finally, in 2010 a Democratic-controlled Congress passed, and President Obama signed, the Affordable Care Act. At the time, Congress told us the "crisis" was that 16 percent of Americans lacked health insurance. So critical was this crisis, that Congress decided to overhaul the entire health care finance system and center its regulation and oversight in Washington, D.C. Since then, the real crisis, the one each individual American has been forced to confront, has really become apparent – out-of-control cost of health insurance.

If politicians were honest about their reform efforts during the past six decades, they would drop the term "health care" and use the right term – health care finance, better known as "insurance." They would admit that their reform efforts are directed at prodding trillions of dollars out of Americans for health "insurance," and using those trillions to construct a massive, expensive bureaucracy run by MediCrats.

Rigged: How Insurance Ruined Health Care

ACA reformers, however, didn't totally ignore the cost of care – they tried to control it through squeezing insurance company revenues using many tools. The Medical Loss Ratio is one of those tools.

Congress decided that insurance companies would be limited to 20 percent of the total premium they collected to pay all their administrative and marketing cost for fully-insured individual and small-group employer health plans. For large employer group insurance, those over 100 employees, the reformers ordered insurance carriers to get by on 15 percent. Politicians believed that by controlling an insurance company's net revenue from premiums, it would slow down health care spending and reduce the price of care. How has that worked out?

Trying to reduce spending and the price of health care services by limiting how much the insurance company can retain is the tail wagging the dog. It required managed-care MediCrats above, outside, and inside each insurance company to try to control spending. It's as if they meant for insurance companies to push the spending boulder up the hill, but do nothing to reduce the size of the boulder.

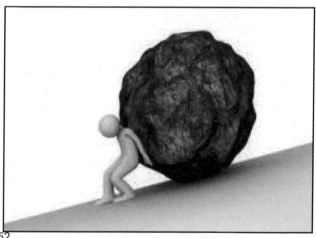

As their vain attempts to force insurance MediCrats to reduce spending continue to fail, politicians answer by once again reforming health finance laws to attempt to shrink the 15 percent to 14 percent -- making the boulder-pusher smaller. This approach cannot possibly control health care cost or spending. When the guy pushing the boulder gets too small, he gets rolled over.

MediCratical Tricks

To control cost, the price of care, and total spending, politicians do have tricks up their sleeve attempting to chip away at the size of the boulder. Their attempt is vintage MediCratical. Congress, either directly or indirectly, imposed controls on medical professionals to force them to provide less care for less money. These controls include the creating of Accountable Care Organizations (ACO), imposition of algorithmic medicine, Big Data, reimbursement incentives, forced compliance with thousands of pages of regulations, and more of the same. Providing medical care has grown more expensive each day as government-imposed regulations increase in number and complexity.

Turning to technology, reformers claim, is a key to reducing spending. Artificial intelligence and crunching a massive volume of data inputs is their hope. Ironically, however, time has shown that as technology improves, total spending goes up, not down.

Many older folks remember holding a personal, palm-sized electronic calculator in their hands for the first time in the 1960s. Most, however, could not afford one when it first became available. Texas Instruments' earliest versions could cost as much as $200, so total spending on hand-held, electronic calculators was miniscule. Within several years, however, technology exploded resulting in a handheld calculator that everyone could own for $20 or $10. Total spending on electronic calculators, with prices slashed 90 percent, spiked higher simply because millions of people bought them.

Today we remember the late 1990s, when flat-screen TVs first appeared on the market. Price tags usually exceeded $4,000, and created civil strife as couples fought over the need to replace their 24" console color TVs. Since their introduction, however, prices have plummeted. On "Black Friday 2016," if you arrived early enough at your local discount store, you could find an Element 43" Smart UHD TV for $199.99, and in some places, there were even better deals. Today, many households have two, three, or more TVs, and total national spending on them has skyrocketed – more people buying more TVs at a reduced price.

The supply of health care services available to any single individual today is mind-boggling. In many ways, technology has made this possible. Whereas 50 years ago, heart attacks and strokes were nearly always fatal, today's technology allows a medical professional to peer into arteries and veins, and see problems before or as they are developing. This ability to see inside the body increases the number of corrective prescribed procedures, even if done a reduced price, so that overall health care spending increases.

Undetected cancer takes the lives of millions of people each year. Technology, however, allows physicians to discover cancer cells at their earliest stage of development. Now able to spot the tiniest hidden cancer cells means more hope for a successful treatment, longer life, and hopefully, will reduce pain and suffering. The price of cancer intervention can be enormous, whether it's the latest drugs or devices that result from cutting-edge research.

Mayo Clinic spent $180 million on one three-story building in Rochester, Minnesota and a second one in Arizona. The new technology housed in this building will provide Mayo's medical professionals with the ability to perform a very precise, specific radiological procedure in the hopes of curing cancer and extending life. "In properly selected patients – especially children and young adults and those with cancers located close to critical organs and body structures – proton beam therapy is an advance over traditional radiotherapy."[2] When the new proton beam therapy facility opened in May 2015, Mayo Clinic announced its hope to serve as many as 138 patients a day – expensive but effective. As Mayo Clinic masters this technology and fills its treatment suite with patients, the cost per procedure will go down, but total spending for the procedure will increase, and the patients, who would have otherwise died, will spend hundreds of thousands more on health care during their extended lives.

To slow down the increase in health care spending, government reformers could prohibit new, cutting-edge technology like proton beam therapy. On the other hand, without health insurance to pay the cost, if individuals had control of their health care dollars, the procedure might be made less expensive.

New drugs and procedures, then, can drive down the price of care, but result in an increase in overall spending, simply because more people have access to more care for more years of their life.

But at What Price?

Diagnostic technology – MRI, MRA, PET Scans, CAT Scans, Ultrasound, X-Rays, etc. – makes it possible for physicians to identify the tiniest threat to a person's life and as a result, prescribe a precision procedure to correct it. Each

---

[2] Staff. "Mayo Clinic Launches Proton Beam Therapy Program." Mayo Clinic. Accessed May 23, 2017. http://mayoclinic.org.

procedure adds to the total number of procedures done each year and results in increased health care spending across the system.

Health plan MediCrats often require a physician to get permission (pre-authorization) to use diagnostic technology on a patient. MediCrats believe many physicians waste money prescribing these procedures (the MediCrats' goal: to spend less on less care).

Diagnostic tests, even when done by the same equipment for the same purpose, can vary in price by 200-2,000 percent. In some communities, Medibid.com can find an MRI for as little as $250, while a hospital across the street will charge $5,000. Remarkably, the test results might be read and interpreted by the same radiologist who works in a lab separate from both entities. It may be that the third-party payer will only allow the hospital to be paid $1,250 instead of $5,000 (a 75 percent "discount"), but even so, the payer will spend $1,250 instead of $250. The reason? The health plan hides the true cost of a procedure from the insured person, and the insured person has no incentive to care about cost. Why?

If Jenny owns a traditional individual health plan, she may pay a $50 co-pay for the MRI, while the insurance company pays another $1,200. The $1,200, in theory, translates into a $1,500 premium, when allowing for the 20 percent of premium the insurance company can retain based on federal law. Jenny's exorbitant and nearly unaffordable insurance premiums, which gave her the "privilege" of only paying $50 for her MRI, result from the interference of the third-party payer system in determining a price point for MRIs – and all other services.

What if Jenny's employer used Medibid.com instead of a traditional health plan? Instead of a $1,500 cost to the health plan for the MRI, the plan would pay $250, the price

Medibid.com found and to which the diagnostic center agreed, for Jenny's test. Instead of using a PPO and spending $1,500, the employer's health plan would turn to Medibid.com and spend $250. The author is aware of one employer who used this concept to reduce his annual health plan cost from over $2 million to less than $800,000 – a 60 percent reduction.

An MRI provider cannot say no to Jenny, although the third-party payer may deny preauthorization for the service. Yet, only Jenny can say no.

The medical professionals in Jenny's PPO network are subject to their reimbursement contracts, and there is a wide range of payment amounts that vary from contract to contract. Jenny has nothing to do with writing or negotiating these contracts – she just pays premiums. She has no skin in the game.

If Jenny had no insurance, a reference-based payment plan, a membership in a health care sharing ministry, or a Health Savings Account (HSA), would motivate Jenny to be more concerned about paying a fair price for her MRI. Jenny would ask the doctor why the test was necessary, and then shop for the best price.

Jenny, and her husband Jerry, recently moved to a new apartment. The living room had beautiful wood floors, but Jenny preferred carpeting. From time-to-time, she would look at rugs in an import shop near her apartment building. One day she saw THE rug – a gorgeous wool import in just the right colors. The salesperson said, "We've discounted it by 50 percent," as Jenny looked at the $14,300 net price. Not owning a prepaid "rug-purchasing plan," Jenny realized she'd be on the hook for the entire $14,300. "I love it," she said, "but my budget won't allow it." She left the store.

Later that day, while buying groceries at a discount store, she saw several area rugs in the Housewares Department, rolled out in a huge stack on the display floor. Inexpensive nylon rugs though they were, Jenny saw one that would work. "$169," she sighed. "That fits my budget." Jenny had her rug, and also held onto more of her cash.

Health plans really do not have a maximum spending budget. They do have targets created by actuaries and accountants, but these are not based on an individual's spending experience. The projected spending is based on a pool of plan members, how much they spend in a year on health care services. The health plan, according to the ACA, must budget 80 percent of premium dollars to pay for covered services, and can retain 20 percent for its overhead expenses (85 and 15 percent for large group health plans). The health plan pools together its best estimate of the total it thinks all its premium-payers (usually called members) will spend in a year, adds its allowable MLR percentage, and determines what it hopes is the maximum the group will spend. The insurance company actuaries understand that the rule of large numbers means they can at least attempt to pinpoint a target spending number for the group. All that is left is to divide the total spend, including overhead costs, by the expected number of members to arrive at a premium amount.

The ACA prohibited setting an annual or lifetime limit on claims for any individual covered by a health plan. Politicians knew that very few people understand health care financing, or why an insurance plan should limit the total dollars that could be spent. In contrast, individuals who own life insurance understand that it will only pay a death benefit up to the policy limit. Insured drivers understand that if they "total" their car in a collision, the insurance company will limit payment to the car's cash value. If they suffer bodily harm in the car wreck, their auto insurance will quit paying for care once the total reaches its maximum contracted limit

– the contract is directly with the insured person, not a provider.

People have come to expect something completely different from their health insurance – expecting all spending to be covered, without limit. Since the ACA passed, politicians realize that setting a maximum limit on health insurance spending will cost them reelection. Hence, health plans will pay without limit – no maximum amount per year or a lifetime.

Jenny's husband Jerry developed pneumonia. Between his hospitalization and other related medical expenses, he blew right past the couple's deductible and the maximum $14,300 out-of-pocket limit for which they were responsible. "Sure glad we have that HSA," Jerry said, to help pay the $14,300 even as he tried to figure out the nearly incomprehensible bills sent to him by medical providers. He only wished he had been able to control some of the spending on his care, given that no one told him the cost while he lay in a hospital bed.

Once Jerry recovered from his pneumonia and returned to work, he realized something. From that point on in that insurance year, his health plan would have to pay for every covered service for both Jenny and him. "We've been paying out $1,500 a month in premium all year," Jerry said, "and I think we should take care of all the medical needs we can now. What do you think?"

"Well I think we have the right to use it," Jenny exclaimed!

"You've been complaining about your sore knees," he said to Jenny that evening, "so I think you should go get it checked out. And I'm going to get that surgery done to fix the hernia on my navel." Jerry realized that, unlike Jenny's decision not to spend $14,300 on a rug, the couple had already spent that much on health care – and at least for that year, and they had no more spending limits, because someone else would have to pay their way.

Jerry also saw a sleep specialist. When the Physician Assistant recommended a CPAP for sleep apnea, Jerry never asked the price.

Jenny had surgery to fix a minor tear in her meniscus. She never asked the price. They had no budget maximum.

At least in theory, the two could demand that the health plan pay out an infinite number of dollars for covered care that year. In many ways, the insurance company did not have to care about the total Jenny and Jerry spent because it raised the premiums the following year for everyone in their "pool" to cover it. In fact, the following year, Jerry and Jenny considered dropping their coverage when they saw their premium increase by 11 percent.

With traditional health insurance, both the policy owner and the medical provider are incentivized to spend more, not less, especially once the out-of-pocket maximum has been passed. If anything, they are trying to cement more dollars to the health spending boulder as it threatens to roll over and destroy health care finance.

Many Americans who discuss health care really are talking about health plans – health insurance. Yet "health" insurance is also a misnomer. A health insurance policy is designed to provide money when a person becomes sick, even though we often talk of wellness or preventive care. The fact is that wellness and preventive care are cheap compared to life-saving surgery, cancer treatment, or the cost of treating chronic disease. Just as life insurance, which only pays a benefit upon death, does not help you live longer, neither does health insurance make you healthier – it pays when you get sick or injured.

Rigged: How Insurance Ruined Health Care

The only way to combat the upward trend in health care spending is for the patient to be in control of spending, with skin in the game.

When it's your money

Jenny owned a 10-year old car because it fit her budget. She meant to keep it running for as many years as possible, because she had learned the lesson that the "cheapest car you will ever own is the one you own." To save money, she dropped collision coverage from her auto insurance policy, saving her more than $600 a year in premiums.

One day, while Jenny backed her old car out of a tight parking spot, she got too close to a wall and dented her rear quarter panel, scraping off some paint. Since the car had already started to rust, she felt certain it needed to be repaired. "How much is this going to cost me?" she asked Al, the auto body repairman.

Al carefully inspected the damage and went inside, where he punched numbers into a computer. "Well, it looks like we can do this for $1,250," he said, smiling at her. "It will look like new when I'm done. Can I have your insurance card?"

Jenny felt faint. "Okay. I don't have collision insurance. So, how much if you pound out the dent, fill it with Bondo, and spray some paint on it?" Jenny had a budget because she had to write the entire check for the repair. She agreed to pay $625 for the repair.

She told the story to her best friend Jackie later that day. "Oh Al gives fair prices. I had almost the same damage on my car, and only had to pay $500 for the deductible. Al got me a new fender, new wheel, new chrome, and repainted half the car. My insurance paid the rest."

Jenny wanted to pay as little as possible for her car insurance. She didn't worry about pushing a boulder uphill. Instead, she bought a few pebbles of necessary coverage and stuck within her budget for the fender repair.

Get us the biggest discount

Grant Jones had called on the procurement officer in Big Buck County for several years in a row. Grant hoped to become their insurance agent of record, and as a resident of the county, he also wanted to save taxpayers' money. He had done his homework, and he knew the county paid at least 35 percent more for their employee health plan than necessary.

Since Big Buck County is a government agency, the procurement office must seek bids each year as it renews its health plan. Grant kept an eye on the Requests for Proposals and went into action as soon as the county posted it on its website.

Grant did his homework. He devised three different health plans with average monthly premiums of about $625 per employee per month, while heeding the plan's design requirements as expressed in the Request For Proposal (RFP). The insurance companies, however, seemed to be cavalier about the bids they provided him, though no one told him about the county's preference.

"Well Mr. Jones, these are real good premiums you've shown me here," the procurement officer said after looking at his proposal. He kept searching the documents and seemed confused. "I can't find the discounts you won us in this proposal," he said.

"Discounts? Well, they are substantial. I didn't document it but I know they are 50 percent or more," Grant answered, scratching his head.

"Well I am very sorry Mr. Jones," the officer said, "but

your plan isn't even close to the broker we have used for many years. He's won us a 75 percent discount from the providers," the officer said, "and we're going to renew with him again this year." Standing up, he shook Jones' hand and said, "Better luck next year."

The procurement officer never realized the other insurance broker's discount was based on an inflated price. "Sure, we can give you a 75 percent discount," the insurance company representative said. Both plans paid the physician $65 for an office visit, but in one case, it was a 50 percent "discount" from $130, and in the other, a 75 percent discount from $260. The insurance company had negotiated a reimbursement for an office visit with its PPO member providers at $65. The retail price really didn't much matter, except that the larger discount looked better on paper. Unfortunately for the county, one element of the plan charges a percentage of the savings, so the plan with a 75 percent discount from $260 would cost more than the 50 percent discount from $130.

Do not discount this story. It is based on an actual case with which the author is familiar. The county had bought into the idea that discounts meant more than the premium they paid to access them. Truly, confusion reigns when it comes to health plan pricing.

In Chapter 11, we explain reference-based payment health insurance plans. We are convinced that these are a better way to price and pay for health care services than relying on the expensive third-party, PPO/HMO system to which we've grown accustomed.

What's Your Reference?

When Jenny shopped for an area rug, she knew how much she could pay for it. The maximum price had to fit her budget. The price she could pay is her reference price. The importer also had a reference price - $14,300. He may have been willing to negotiate a lesser price if Jenny had been willing to pay more. Perhaps he would have accepted $9,995. But Jenny knew she could not stretch much beyond $300. Both parties agreed there would be no deal between them.

While the complexities of health care make it nearly impossible to have a "best" way to pay for care, a reference-based payment system will work for most people in most situations. It could overcome many obstacles to making wise decisions about the need for care and the price to which the payer and provider will agree.

Reference-priced payments help overcome the moral hazard posed by third-party payer systems in which providers and payers are each trying to get as much out of the system as possible. With third-party systems, the patient feels as though they are not getting value unless they spend money in the system, and the physician only gains when the patient uses insurance, but will lose in the long run doing more than necessary. In a reference-based payment system, each party always has skin in the game and it brings balance to the decision about consuming medical care.

Jenny and Jerry went to dinner with Ralph and Rhonda. As they enjoyed their dinner and conversation, no one asked about who would pay the bill. Jenny preferred each couple paying their own way. Jerry loved to pay the bill as a matter of pride. Ralph quietly agreed with Jenny, while Rhonda felt nervous, just knowing they would have to make a decision eventually.

Finally, Jerry said, "Hey, we will get this," as he picked up the black folder with the bill in it.

"I wish I would have ordered the lobster," Ralph said, as Rhonda poked him hard in the ribs. Ralph might have been joking, but this does reveal a small piece of human nature – we like spending other peoples' money and when we do, we are not always careful.

The biggest threat to health care is the third-party payment system, its networks, and blind spending by patients that drive overconsumption and overspending. This is how insurance is ruining health care.

Rigged: How Insurance Ruined Health Care

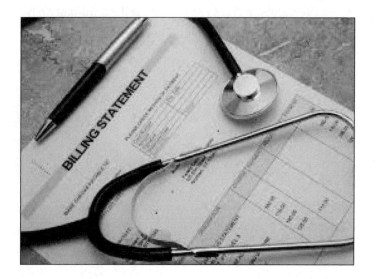

Chapter 11

Key to True Consumerism - Reference-Based Payment

Except for the "rent seekers"[1] who profit by the complexity of health care finance, almost everyone at least pays lip service to the idea that patients should be able to see the price of the care they receive before receiving it. This is generally called price transparency. "If someone only knew what it costs, they'd make better decisions," some folks reason. This can be true, if the patient is empowered with the right plan, the right tools to make it possible, and sufficiently motivated to care about it.

Health care reformers commonly say that care should be focused on the patient, not the payment system. Patients, however, have been left little, if any recourse about the price of care. They never see the real price of care until after the fact, yet cannot make informed spending decisions without seeing it.

---

[1] **Rent seeking** is a predatory practice where an outsider siphons value out of an economic process—yet provides little or no value to the actual participants. *Rent seekers* are unneeded middlemen." Danby, J. (2016) *Common Sense Medicine.* Alethos Press. St. Paul, MN. 2016. P 8.

Furthermore, once the patient has paid the annual deductible and exceeded the out-of-pocket maximum, the patient has no more "skin in the game," and has little incentive to be an informed consumer. In fact, the author has seen cases where transparency increases spending. Allow me to illustrate:

> Joe owns a health plan with a $6,000 deductible. He needs a knee replacement and is offered two different orthopedic surgeons. The first surgeon charges $18,000, the second charges $95,000 for the same procedure. Joe looks at the two prices and (mistakenly) takes the charges as a proxy for quality, and given the same $6,000 deductible, he selects the more expensive surgeon.

Learning the price after the fact
A sure way to pay too much

More than 89 percent of medical care consumed today is paid for by a third-party[2] – usually a government agency (directly or indirectly), insurance company, or employer. The patient, if he or she ever does, will not learn the actual price paid for his or her care until receiving an Explanation of Benefits (EOB), weeks and sometimes months later.

Moreover, the medical professional or facility providing the care will not know how much they will be paid until they receive the Explanation of Payment (EOP) from a third-party payer. Unless the payer makes a contractual mistake, the medical professional is unlikely to contest the amount of the payment.

Third-party payers use a contract to lock in the amount they agree to pay the medical professional. During contract negotiations, medical professionals set their retail price at an

---

[2] CMS. *National Health Expenditures – Historical*. 2016.

Rigged: How Insurance Ruined Health Care

unreasonably high level – and then the third-party payer "discounts" it. (This is called the Chargemaster System – see Chapter 6.) The EOB shows how much the health plan will pay of the total bill, and since providers are used to the payer applying a "discount," they are usually happy to at least receive partial payment. Occasionally the provider may "balance bill" the patient, so appropriate shopping tools need to be built into the plan. At the end of the EOB, the patient will finally see how much he or she must pay.

The amount the patient will pay depends on his or her health plan contract. He may pay a co-payment at the time of service, followed by his share of the deductible. Eventually, if he needs a good deal of medical care, he will exceed the maximum out-of-pocket payments specified in his health plan contract. Once he exceeds his maximum out-of-pocket share in a year, he throws off all spending restraint and seeks even more care. All the time he is "buying" these services he never knows the price of care until after the fact. No other economic system operates in this fashion.

One might expect that employers with self-funded health plans are particularly careful about how much they pay for the medical care received by their employees – this is not so. Like the individual who receives an EOB, the employer's plan administrator will seldom if ever have a clue about the real price of care.

> [The plan administrator will] … receive a useless Uniform Bill (UB) from a hospital as an invoice, they deduct the PPO discount from the billing and they pay with someone else's money. There is absolutely nothing on a UB that allows the [patient] to know what is being billed for nor the accuracy of those billings.[3]

---

[3] Chase, Dave. "Have PPO Networks Perpetrated The Greatest Heist In American History?" *Forbes*, September 5, 2016. http://www.forbes.com/sites/davechase/2016/09/05/have-ppo-networks-perpetrated-the-great-

The plan administrator pays the bill, and gets on with her day. The company frets about increased cost of the health plan, but renews it each year, preferring to focus on their primary business mission.

For all intents and purposes, every employer in America gives every covered member on their healthcare plan a blank check every year and says....consume all the healthcare you want, anywhere you want, anytime you want, and never be concerned with or ask the price because it's all paid for.[4]

The fact that employers provide near carte blanch payment for medical care spent by their employees runs contrary to how they run their business. Most successful businesses have established a budget that brings discipline to spending and limits any payments beyond the budgeted amount. Yet, they do not do this with health care payments under their self-insured programs, instead, relying on third-parties to watch their spending for them, and send them the bill.

Preferred Provider Organizations (PPO)
People like them, but they are expensive

Most Americans love the idea of someone setting up a provider organization for them. It simplifies their search for a doctor or hospital, or other medical care – but patients pay a steep price for this service and it directly contributes to the increasingly unaffordable health "insurance" plans they hope to purchase. Instead of cherishing the freedom to choose their own doctor or hospital, however, he or she seems to prefer the simplicity of looking at a provider direc-

---

est-heist-in-american-history/.
[4] Ibid.

tory and setting an appointment. They need a different, better, more responsible way to choose a doctor.

The PPO system dates to the early 1970s as a move away from fee-for-service medicine, and has become deeply ingrained in America. The PPO confuses the discussion about patient choice. In a PPO, the patient's choice is essentially limited to the providers with whom a third-party has signed a contract. It's like the old adage about Model T Fords – "You can have your choice of color, as long as it is black."

The fact that a doctor is in a network is not a proxy for quality. Yet most often, patients chose their doctor because he appears first in the directory. Therefore, a patient is more likely to choose Dr. Adams than Dr. Smith, and they assume Dr. Adams is competent and qualified.

Under the PPO delivery model, someone else is paid to organize the individual's health care and sets the price of care, without consulting the policy-owner. The insured pays "rent" in the form of monthly premiums, over which he or she has very little control. After Congress passed the Affordable Care Act in 2010, the individual's share of their medical bill, in the form of premiums, deductibles and out-of-pocket expenses, has skyrocketed. All this time, however, he or she has had no control over the price of care.

The Monroney Sticker Price

When you walk into an auto showroom, after being dazzled by the stylish sports car or enticed by the luxury town car, you find the sticker on the window. You examine the sticker price and see all the various charges that have been added to the factory price – delivery, preparation, dealer-added features, etc. If you purchase the car you will probably not pay the sticker price – the dealer may offer a discount, or provide other incentives – but at least you know the price before you start the buying process.

The sticker price on a car is the result of the perseverance of United States Senator Almer Stillwell Monroney, an Oklahoma Democrat. Monroney, the chief sponsor of the 1958 bill that mandated automobile sticker prices, saw this as a way to increase honest competition by dealers.

> "The dealer who is honest about the so-called 'list price' cannot compete with the one who 'packs' several hundred dollars extra into it so he can pretend to give you more on your trade-in," Monroney said when the bill was introduced in March 1958.[5]

Perhaps today's Congress should mandate that all medical procedures must show a Reference-Price Sticker that details the cost of care, so the patient can make informed decisions before care is provided. At MediBid.com, a patient receives just that – a price in advance which holds for the procedures, baring complications or misstatement.

What if you knew the price?

Knowing the price of care before receiving it would make an individual a health care consumer, not just a user (or worse, an abuser). Then he or she can ask the medical professional, "Why do I need this?" "How much does this cost?," "What are my options?" Knowing the price of care, and having reason to be concerned about it, puts him or her in charge of their own lives. This is what real choice in health care looks like – the patient is in control.

Granted, when a serious illness suddenly occurs, or an individual suffers an accident or injury, he or she often does

---

[5] Peele, Robert. "The Senator Behind the Window Sticker." *The New York Times*, January 2, 2009. http://www.nytimes.com/2009/01/04/automobiles/04MONRONEY.html.

not have time to worry about the price of care. All she wants is medical attention, now! But the prudent health care consumer can research prices ahead of time and have a good idea of where to seek care, if she is able to do so.

There is, however, another way to know the price of care, and have control over it. It is commonly known as reference-based pricing, although reference-based payment is a more accurate term.

> Reference-based reimbursement [pricing] is the most straightforward path that hundreds of companies have proven can be implemented rapidly to save the American Dream. ... it is saving schools, businesses and municipalities millions every year — money that can end the economic depression for the middle class if it isn't redistributed from the middle class to an administratively bloated industry paying executives fabulous salaries for average performance (from a health outcomes perspective).[6]

Well-designed reference-based payment plans can reduce an individual's health care costs by over 35 percent. Those are savings worth exploring, if the plan is properly designed and easy to use.

In general, a reference-based payment system, unlike a PPO/HMO/ACO traditional pricing system, works in this manner – the plan either pays the medical professional a set reference price or a percentage above a reference price.

The most widely used pricing scale for the greatest volume of medical care is the price Medicare sets to pay a medical professional. (Medicare does not pay for all types of services for all types of people – maternity benefits for example, or pediatric care – but there are other set pricing systems that can be used as reference prices for those.)

---

[6] See Chase, Note 3.

John and Jane Smith purchase a new, reference-based pricing plan that pays a medical provider 50 percent above Medicare's reimbursement. John's physician has set her chargemaster price for a physical at $600, but she knows that the Medicare price is only $165. Her average reimbursement from an insurance company is $280.

John presents the physician with his Medicare-reference-priced plan, which offers to pay $165 times 150 percent, or $247.50. The physician has to make a decision. Should she settle for $247.50, which is still far more than she would receive for a Medicare patient, or should she balance bill the patient?

To balance bill means charging the difference between what the plan will pay and what the medical professional will accept. John's doctor might ask him for an additional $32.50, or even $352.50 (in which case, John will likely find a different physician). The choice over the balanced billing amount is a negotiation between John and his physician. They will decide, not a government agency or a third-party payer.

John's plan is administered by a third-party, but under his control. He decides whether to accept the physician's price or go shopping. The physician decides whether to accept the referenced price, or charge more.

Under John's plan, he may still have a co-pay or a deductible. The plan can be designed in a number of ways. The critical factor is that it requires transparent pricing and shopping tools before John decides whom to hire as his physician.

This simplified example, where John seeks a price

that fits his Medicare-plus reference-priced health plan, will work for all non-emergency medical care. For surgical procedures that do not have to be done immediately, it is particularly valuable.

CALPERS, the California health plan for state employees, has set a price it is willing to pay for total knee replacements at about $30,000. In other words, $30,000 is its reference-based price for total knee replacements, and as a result, most California facilities charge $30,000. It is possible that if Jane Smith needs a total knee replacement, her Medicare-plus health plan, which pays 50-percent over Medicare, will only allow $17,000. What can Jane do? She can go shopping.

Using MediBid, Jane will let the orthopedic surgeons who compete for business on MediBid.com know about her surgical need. From experience, it is likely she will find the same surgical procedure in a nearby state – or even in California – for a price easily within the limits of her Medicare-plus plan.

Better yet, if John and Jane receive their Medicare-plus plan from their employer, the employer may be willing to pay the travel expenses involved, and a bonus for saving the plan some money. The key factor in all this is the ability to ascertain the price of the knee replacement from a competent, professional surgeon in a quality facility ahead of time. Knowing that the health plan pays only up to a certain limit creates the negotiating pressure between Jane and the surgeon and his facility.

Reference-based pricing plans, like the Medicare-plus-a-percent concept, could eliminate the need for a PPO, and save the patient and physician the added cost of letting the PPO control access to medical care, while adding its "rental" fees – a per member per month processing fee, and sometimes even a "percentage of savings" – to the bill.

Rigged: How Insurance Ruined Health Care
Any Willing Provider

John and Jane Smith, with their reference-based pricing plan, are freed from the constraints and prohibitive cost of a PPO. They can purchase – hire, if you think about it – any willing medical professional to provide their care. Not only can they choose which physician they hire or facility they use, they can also choose to fire that provider, and yet, their reference-based payment plan still provides them with financial security and protection against bankruptcy.

Not all medical professionals or facilities will accept the Medicare-plus payments as paying in full for their services. Some will balance-bill, and this can be more of a threat for emergency services. It should be the right of a medical professional to set his or her own fees. If they prefer to charge more than the plan will pay, the patient will make a decision based on perceived value. If the patient values that particular physician enough, he or she will pay the balance. If not, he or she will go shopping.

When John and Jane inquire about receiving care from a new physician or facility, they will ask whether their Medicare-plus plan will provide sufficient payment to the provider - and many physicians would jump at the chance of receiving payment this way. If the provider will not accept the Medicare-plus rate, the Smiths will continue their search. It puts the decision in the hands of the patient and doctor, not a third-party payer.

The Smiths' Medicare-plus plan has been modified with an attractive option, however, to pay up to 200 percent of Medicare's rate for emergency services. This feature allows the Smiths more security, knowing that should something out of their control happen, their financial risk is reduced.

If the Smiths receive care from a physician or facility

that balance bills and demands payments, there is a potential solution. The Smiths could call a "repricer," a service-provider that negotiates on behalf of the Smiths. The repricer will negotiate a settlement with the provider, and both parties know the limits of this negotiation. There is settled litigation[7] on a reasonable price for what medical services ought to cost, and if possible, no one really wants to go to court to win a settlement that neither side can accept.

The reference-pricing system will work best when patients cannot only find the reference price, but also find medical professionals and facilities willing to accept that reference price with no balanced billing. It is even better when the patient can find a price below the reference price. The reality is that pre-negotiated or posted pricing may not yield the best results if the provider sets a price just below the reference price but the patient doesn't know about it. Medical bidding services, such as MediBid.com, can always yield the best results, as providers compete for a patient's business.

Think of four gas stations sitting on four corners of the same intersection. Each day the stations post their price per gallon, and sometimes, when they see their competitor's price, they raise or reduce their own price. Open and transparent pricing between competitors generally results in the best price to fill up your gas tank.

Health care services, pharmaceuticals, and medical device pricing can, likewise, be subjected to competitive bidding if someone, like MediBid.com, is able to gather those prices for the patient. At MediBid.com, the patient uploads basic information about his or her need, and willing providers bid on it showing him or her not only their price,

---

Rooney, Dan Perrin J. Patrick. *America's Health Care Crisis Solved: Money-Saving Solutions, Coverage for Everyone.* Hoboken, NJ: Wiley, John & Sons, Incorporated, 2008.[7]

but also their educations, training, experience, quality and outcomes. At times, MediBid.com calls providers to secure the best possible price. This price-shopping service augments the patient's power to maximize the value of their Medicare-plus, referenced-based pricing health plan.

The power of competitive pricing tends to drive the price lower while improving quality, when true transparency is achieved and published.

Lesson Learned

Early in his career, the author worked as an administrator for the AAA in Canada (CAA). Among his duties, he oversaw the payment of towing charges. At the beginning, the CAA paid a towing company $20.00 for a tow within a specified radius, and $1.25 more per kilometer if the tow exceeded the basic radius.

The author noticed that the average towing fees exceeded $27. The towing companies believed that the amount was too small to merit much audit from the CAA, which would simply pay the bill. This billing method encouraged creative billing – cheating.

At this point, the author polled all towing companies, noting that the average tow was 11 KM. He said, "If we pay you a flat fee per tow, how much will you accept in payment for tows within city limits?" In this manner, he let each towing company set its own price, or "bid." After launching his new pricing plan based on what the towing companies said they would accept, he found that his average price settled in at $24. This pricing system reduced CAA's cost and made the system more profitable for all parties, while eliminating cheating and unnecessary, burdensome paperwork.

Many foreign countries with government-run health care systems set the price they are willing to pay for prescription medicines during negotiations with pharmaceutical companies. If the company does not agree to the price the government is willing to pay, then the drug is not made available under the plan. The government-negotiated price is the reference price.

Naturally, there are patent and trade issues involved in the sale of pharmaceuticals and medical devices and supplies. Yet, government-run health systems in foreign nations present a more unified price control system than does the United States and its myriad of health plans. Some countries have learned how to use and abuse international law by declaring a national emergency, such as an outbreak of diabetes, Hepatitis C, a type of cancer, or coronary heart disease. The country then authorizes a company domiciled in its borders to manufacture the drug, thereby saving the government health plan large sums of money.

Reference-based payments allow each provider and payer to always start their negotiation at $0.00 – zero-based budgeting. The pricing starts over each year, and sometimes even for each procedure, under current conditions, from the bottom up – not the top down, at a price dictated by a third-party payer. This system can produce personal choice, better access to care, and a lower cost – the goals reformers say they want to achieve. What is lacking to make this most effective is a resolve by millions of individuals and employers to make the switch.

Simply stated, and easy to understand, if a medical professional sets his or her price for a service, it is a reference price. If a health plan sets a price it will pay for a service, it is a reference price. When both sides choose referencing pricing, a price-point market is created for medical care, and better yet, when the medical professional publishes their prices ahead of time – like a Monroney Sticker – the patient can make an informed decision.

Rigged: How Insurance Ruined Health Care

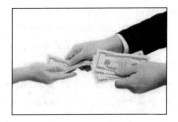

Chapter 12

Sharing Health Care Cost: An American Tradition

The United States spent $3.2 trillion on health care in 2016. The share paid out-of-pocket by individuals was just less than 11 percent of total spending. Third parties paid for 89 percent of this spending. The "rest of the story" about that 89 percent, however, is that individuals, through their taxes, insurance premiums, and higher prices for care, paid 100 percent of the bill.

Since the ACA health plans hit the marketplace in January of 2014, individuals are increasingly becoming aware of the nearly unaffordable health insurance premiums. Tens of thousands of people have begun searching for an alternative to traditional, third-party paid health "insurance."

For a variety of reasons, cost being one critical factor, an increasing number of people are opting for health care sharing ministries (HCSM) as an affordable, alternative way to pay for health care. "At least another 530,000 are enrolled in medical cost-sharing plans, usually run as religious ministries,"[1] stated a February 23, 2016 *U.S. News and World*

---

[1] Beecher, Lee, MD.; Racer, Dave. (2017) *Passion for Patients*. Alethos Press, St. Paul, MN. P 47 (ebook version)

Report article. HCSMs have seen explosive growth – one has seen growth of more than 6,000 percent since 2015.

In Section 5000A(d)2(B) of the ACA, Congress made provision for HCSMs that were in place prior to December 31, 1999. Membership in a HCSM satisfies the individual mandate requirement to maintain minimum essential coverage. Six HCSMs of which the author is aware, meet the requirements of the ACA:

- Samaritan Ministries (1994),
- Christian Healthcare Ministries (1981)
- Christian Care Ministry – Medi-Share (1993)
- Liberty Health Share (1998)
- South East Mennonite Medical Aid Society, Kentucky – SEMMA
- Altrua HealthShare

A number of other small ministries, such as those for Amish and Mennonite members, also qualified.

Other HCSMs have attempted to form since December 31, 1999, and claim they qualify under the law. However some of them do not. Potential enrollees should be very careful about signing up with groups not included in the above list, and ask to see written proof from the Centers for Medicare and Medicaid Services (CMS) that the plan qualifies under the law.

The long track record of the established HCSMs is also an important consideration, since for them to function well, they need the experience to provide good counsel for their enrollees as they deal with providers who are not used to the sharing ministry's terms.

At least three of these HCSMs require that the applicant sign a statement of personal Christian faith, attested to by a pastor or priest. These groups openly espouse Biblical principles of burden-sharing and how these principles apply to payment for care and other membership criteria. The ministries encourage members to pray for and encourage each other – "bearing each other's burdens."[2] Two HCSMs, Liberty and Altrua, do not have religious tests, but rather allow for "ethical" tests, and are allowed under the ACA definition of a Health Care Sharing Ministry.

HCSMs generally do not accept individuals with pre-existing conditions. In most cases, smokers and obese persons are not allowed to enroll. At least one HCSM has a special provision for some otherwise unhealthy members who are accepted in a health track program and agree to cease smoking and engage in a weight-loss plan – these individuals will pay a greater fee. Once a person is enrolled as a regular member in these HCSMs, however, they will remain so. The HCSM does not force them out because of a subsequent illness or accident.

Not insurance

Health Care Sharing Ministries are not insurance. They are exactly what the term says – sharing the cost of health care services. Members share the cost of paying for each other's medical bills. Monthly cost shares are determined based on the HCSM's history of the cost of sharing, and most often, increases in share cost are voted on by ministry members.

Some HCSMs allow members to share all their medical bills after they have met their Annual Household Portion (AHP), or Annual Unshared Amount (AUA). Once the AHP or AUA has been reached, the HCSM will pay the bills, based on their agreement. Each member knows in advance the amount of share the HCSM will pay – and some HCSMs

---

[2] Galatians 6:2. *The Bible.*

pay 100 percent after the AHP or AUA has been reached. This is something like a deductible.

Some HCSMs have a set dollar amount the member must pay before the HCSM will pay, which acts something like a co-pay. This might be as much $300 for each incident that a member will pay directly for their medical care. The HCSM may also set a maximum of payments per year where the member pays the first $300 after which the HCSM will pay the remaining costs.

Each ministry carefully lists the services for which members will share costs and those costs that do not qualify. Some common exclusions are vision, dental, infertility expenses, preventive care, injuries or illness related to commission of a crime, STD treatment, childbirth to an unwed mother, and abortion.

Generally, members of these HCSMs pay a monthly fee based on age and the number of family members. Some of the ministries match an enrollee's monthly fees with the expenses of other members, and disclose who is receiving the benefit, while encouraging the members to pray for each other.

While monthly fees vary between HCSMs, for illustration purposes here, an HCSM may have a monthly fee for a single person of $200 a month, with a $500 annual out-of-pocket limit. A family cost might be $450 a month with a maximum out-of-pocket annual amount of $1,500. HCSMs vary as to the monthly membership fee and out-of-pocket limits.

Dealing with Balanced Bills

Since HCSMs' scheduled payment rates may be less than providers want to charge, and since most HCSMs have no provider network, the individual may be subject to "balanced billing." Balanced bills indicate the amount the HCSM will pay the provider and the difference between the provider's chargemaster or "retail" price and what the HCSM allows. For instance, the HCSM may pay $200 for a physical exam, but the physician charges $600 – and balance bills the patient for the $400 difference. (Any person with a typical commercial health plan that receives care out of their PPO network is likely to receive a balanced bill from the provider – so this situation is not unique to HCSMs.) Some of the HCSMs will negotiate away all, or a portion of the balance bill on behalf of their members.

When confronted with an unaffordable balanced bill, an individual can work with a health care "repricer." For a fee, usually a share of the savings, the repricer will negotiate a settlement with the provider and payment terms for the individual. These repriced services can be dramatically lower than the chargemaster price demanded by the provider. Several HCSMs retain repricers on behalf of their members.

The best way to avoid a balanced bill is for the individual to negotiate the price of care in advance. Almost all medical care can be purchased this way – except for accidents and illnesses that require emergency services. Using a service like MediBid.com can help avoid a balanced bill after the service has been provided, and eliminate the need for a repricer after the fact.

In choosing an HCSM, you will want to know its sharing guidelines and costs in advance. Costs with any given HCSM may be much higher if that HCSM tries to use insurance-like tools (i.e. PPO Network, see Chapter 7) in an attempt to offer convenience to members.

Can employers use HCSMs?

(As this book goes to press, the Affordable Care Act

is still the law of the land. Congress may eliminate the penalties and fines associated with the ACA, and that could open up more opportunities for employers to use health care sharing as an employee benefit. This section, however, addresses the ACA-regulated marketplace.)

As stated earlier in this chapter, health care sharing ministries and health insurance are two separate concepts.

Membership in a recognized HCSM, as defined by the ACA, satisfies the individual mandate to maintain Minimum Essential Coverage (MEC).

An individual must maintain Minimum Essential Coverage (MEC) to satisfy the ACA's individual mandate. Minimum Essential Coverage means that a health plan must have no annual or lifetime limits and offer about 75 preventive health services, with no individual cost-sharing. A pure, preventive-only MEC plan generally costs between $40 to $60 a month.

If the individual is a member of an HCSM that meets the ACA requirements, they are deemed to have satisfied the MEC requirement and do not have to pay the IRS penalty.

The ACA defines an Applicable Large Employer (ALE) as an employer with 50 or more Full Time Equivalent (FTE) employees. FTE is defined as any number of employees who together work an average of 30 hours a week and 130 hours a month (this is an over-simplification for the purpose of this book). For example, three employees each working 10 hours a week would equal one FTE employee.

Under the ACA, an Applicable Large Employer (ALE) is subject to three fines. The first, up to $1,000 per employee per year, is for willful failure to report the data required by law.

The second penalty, $2,260 in 2017 per employee per year – Sec. 4980H(a) – is sometimes called the "Sledge Hammer Penalty." To avoid this penalty, the employer must offer at least a MEC plan to 95 percent of their full-time employees. The penalty is not applied to the first 30 full-time employees, but to the balance of full-time employees.

The third penalty, $3,390 in 2017 – Sec. 4980H(b) – is often called the "Tack Hammer Penalty." This penalty is assessed if the employer does not offer coverage that meets the 60 percent minimum value test, and/or if the coverage is not affordable. Affordability, in 2017, is defined as the employee not having to contribute more than 9.69 percent of his or her income toward the cost of the benefit.

If the plan is not affordable or does not meet minimum value, then the employee is authorized to go to a government-run insurance exchange and may qualify for premium tax credits. To qualify, the individual's adjusted gross household income will determine what, if any, subsidy is available. In some states, the household income must be between 100 and 400 percent of Federal Poverty Guideline (FPG) income. In other states, those that have expanded Medicaid coverage, the qualifying household incomes are between 138 and 400 percent of FPG.

For employers, a MEC plan offered to at least 95 percent of eligible employees satisfies the ACA's Sledge Hammer Penalty. However, the employer may have some exposure to the Tack Hammer Penalty.

A well-versed, experienced employee benefits specialist will be able to counsel you in reducing or eliminating exposure to the Tack Hammer penalty.

Employees offered a MEC plan may choose their own health care options as they see fit. This may mean that they remain uninsured for major medical needs, or they might buy an individual plan, buy supplemental care, or join a Health Care Sharing Ministry (HCSM).

In summary, this chapter is about Health Care Sharing Ministries, usually the choice of individuals and families

Rigged: How Insurance Ruined Health Care

without employer coverage. Yet it is an option for individuals whose employers offer only a MEC Plan. While it is possible to set up a MEC plan and allow an individual to enroll in a HCSM, it requires the assistance of a highly skilled, knowledgeable insurance broker – do not attempt this on your own.

About Ralph Weber

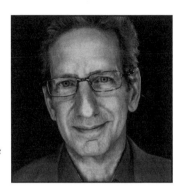

Ralph Weber is a health care consultant, based out of Houston, Texas. Ralph advises self-insured employers, Health Care Sharing Ministries, and foreign governments on how to improve quality and reduce the cost of medical care.

Canadian by birth, Ralph moved to the United States in 2005 when he and his family sought access to better health care than they experienced in Canada. Ralph travels across the United States speaking about Canadian health care, U.S. health care reform, and more affordable ways to finance medical care.

Given his personal experiences in the Canadian health care system, Ralph provides unique and informed insights about government-run medical care. He has a great concern about how the U.S. is moving toward more federal "MediCratic" control of health care.

In 2009, Ralph and a group of investors launched MediBid.com, an online service that matches patients with physicians and surgeons, offering individuals and employers significant improvement in quality, as well as dollar savings on a wide range of health care services. Ralph serves as President of MediBid, Inc.

Ralph has developed and presented numerous teaching programs concerning medical care finance and alternative payment systems. In 2011, Ralph wrote his first book, *MediCrats: Medical Bureaucrats that Rule your Health Care* (revised 2013).[1]

To contact Ralph Weber:

Ralph Weber
403 W Grand Parkway South, Ste F-401
Katy, TX 77494
Office: 888-855-MEDI (6334)

Email: ralph@medibid.com

Website for MediBid: http://www.medibid.com
Website for Ralph: http://www.ralphweber.com
See: http://howinsuranceruinedhealthcare.com

---

[1] Weber, Ralph; Racer, Dave. (2013) *MediCrats: Medical Bureaucrats that Rule your Health Care* (second edition). Alethos Press, St. Paul, MN, 2013.

ABOUT DAVE RACER, MLITT

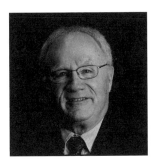

Dave Racer is a Minnesota-based speaker, author, writer, teacher, and publisher. His credits include more than 45 books, 17 of which focus on health care reform in the United States. Other books include true crime, biography, and government.

Dave is a featured speaker on health care reform, America's founding principles, the U.S. Declaration of Independence and Constitution, and contemporary issues.

He is a board member of the Minnesota Physician-Patient Alliance, and the past Legislative Research Director of the Minnesota Association of Health Underwriters.

Dave has a long history of pollical service as a candidate, national presidential campaign manager, writer, and strategist. For six years he hosted *The Dave Racer Show,* a talk radio program in the Twin Cities, and previous to that, published *Dave Racer's Minnesota Report,* a monthly investigative tabloid newspaper.

Dave attended Macalaster College, the University of Minnesota, and the University of Southern Mississippi. He holds a Masters' degree from Oxford Graduate School.

Dave is a U.S. Air Force Veteran.

Rigged: How Insurance Ruined Health Care
To contact Dave Racer:

dgracer@comcast.net

http://www.daveracer.com

http://www.alethospress.com

TO ORDER COPIES OF THIS BOOK:

This book is available in paperback from the author, at Alethos Press, or Amazon.com.

Ralph Weber
403 W Grand Parkway South, Ste F-401
Katy, TX 77494
Office: 888-855-MEDI (6334)

http://www.howhealthinsuranceruinedhealthcare.com

http://www.alethospress.com

http://www.amazon.com

This book is available as a Kindle book at Amazon.com.